19.95

# CLINICAL
# ONCOLOG

D0533632

MRS. JACQUELINE H. OWENS
Toad Hall
Kilburn, York
Yorkshire YO6 4AH
Tel. 034 76 469

# CLINICAL ONCOLOGY

Gareth J.G. Rees MRCP FRCR
Consultant Oncologist, Bristol Radiotherapy and
Oncology Centre and Royal United Hospital, Bath,
UK

**CHP** CASTLE HOUSE PUBLICATIONS

First published in 1989 by
Castle House Publications
Tunbridge Wells, Kent

British Cataloguing in Publication Data

Rees, Gareth, J. G.
    Clinical Oncology.
    1. Oncology
    I. Title
    616.99'2

    ISBN 0-7194-0133-X

Typeset by Keyset Composition, Colchester
Printed and bound in Great Britain by
Billings and Sons Ltd, Worcester

# Contents

# Acknowledgments

I am indebted to several colleagues, especially to Dr Graham Smith, Dr Hugh Newman, Dr Sally Goodman and Dr Edward Gilby, for their corrections and helpful advice.

# Acknowledgements

# Preface

This book is intended as a useful companion to those hospital doctors substantially engaged in the care of adult cancer patients. The emphasis is on the practical aspects of management, but the aim is also to provide a framework for logical decision-making. Some information is provided on specific malignancies so that individual patients may be seen in context, and managed appropriately. There is also a brief introductory chapter on the biology of tumour processes.

The book is divided into two parts. The first part is on general principles and practice, but also includes much detailed information, particularly on drugs and the complications of cancer and its treatment. It is suggested that doctors new to clinical oncology may like to read most of this part early on, omitting some of the finer details. The second part comprises notes on the more common specific cancers. For each malignancy there is an introductory section comprising information on incidence (UK figures), pathology and prognosis. There are then sections on risk factors, symptoms and signs, these being followed by sections on radical and palliative treatments, subdivided by modality. Finally, there are sections on follow-up and 'practice points'.

For reasons of space most rare tumours are excluded, but these notes should be of some relevance to the management of about 95 per cent of cancer patients. There is also very little information on tumour staging and investigations, partly because of lack of space, but also because I have not wished to encourage the concept of 'routine investigations'. Investigations should be requested only if they stand a chance of usefully influencing management.

In places I have given way to personal prejudice and experience and it is inevitable that parts of this book will not present what might be termed a 'consensus view'. I have, however, tried in general to give a balanced viewpoint and would be most grateful if readers would tell me where they think I have failed, or where they discover errors or important omissions.

G.J.G. Rees
Bristol
1989

# PART I

# General Principles and Practice

# CHAPTER 1

# Tumour Biology

## Oncogenes

These are DNA sequences present in normal cell nuclei, and which have the capacity to cause neoplastic change when subjected to influences which result in their altered expression. Normal unaltered oncogenes are known as proto-oncogenes and over thirty different oncogenes have now been identified.

Oncogenesis may take place as a result of abnormally high levels of expression of the unaltered gene (quantitative alteration or 'amplification') or as a result of a mutation which causes the gene to produce a new protein (qualitative alteration). The activation of oncogenes is often associated with chromosomal abnormalities, sometimes of a specific nature, e.g. the 9:22 translocation in chronic granulocytic leukaemia (Philadelphia chromosome) and the 8:2, 14 or 22 translocation in Burkitt's lymphoma, a tumour of B-lymphocytes. In the Burkitt's translocation, the C-myc oncogene is transferred to a chromosomal region which normally codes for immunoglobulins.

Some of the proteins produced by oncogenes in the initiation or maintenance of malignancy have been discovered to have biological effects which may, at least partly, explain the neoplastic process. Some are extremely similar to normal growth factors (e.g. platelet-derived growth factor, epidermal growth factor), or their cell surface receptors. The binding of growth factors to their receptors activates enzymes, such as kinases, and can thereby induce cell division.

As well as their important role in carcinogenesis, oncogenes and their products offer the prospect of assisting in histological diagnosis (immunocytochemistry) and radiodiagnosis (radioimmunoscintigraphy), the assessment of prognosis, and treatment. For example, high levels of the expression of the c-erb oncogene are associated with a particularly poor prognosis in breast cancer patients. Immunocytochemical analysis using monoclonal antibodies directed against oncogene products is feasible on formalin-fixed wax block specimens, and quantitative assessments can be made using flow cytometry. For treatment there is the possibility that monoclonal antibodies linked to toxins or radionuclides may be effectively directed against oncogene products.

## Kinetics

Malignant tumours usually show evidence of increased mitotic activity. Malignant cells do not always multiply faster than their normal counterparts, however, and a tumour results because of an imbalance between cellular proliferation and cell loss. Malignant cells, like normal cells, have a finite life span. A variable proportion of cells within a tumour is malignant and there is often a substantial component of non-malignant stromal or reactive cells. Occasionally, as in lymphocyte-predominant Hodgkin's disease, the proportion of malignant (Reed-Sternberg) cells is extremely small.

Only a proportion of the malignant cells within a cancer has the capacity for indefinite self-replication. These are known as stem cells and are the targets for treatment with radiotherapy or drugs. The proportion of malignant cells proceeding through the cell cycle to mitosis at any one time is known as the growth fraction. The remainder of the malignant cells are in a resting phase and can be recruited into the growth fraction. Conversely, dividing cells may differentiate into mature 'end cells' with no further capacity for proliferation. The growth fraction is sometimes very small indeed but in some rapidly growing tumours it can approach 100 per cent of the total malignant cell population.

The rate of tumour growth depends on the size of the growth fraction and also on the cell cycle time, i.e. the time from one mitosis to the next. The great variations in cellular proliferation and loss account for the very large variation in tumour doubling times, which can vary from a few days to a few years. Initially, the rate of cellular proliferation leads to approximately exponential tumour growth, but subsequently the rate of growth falls off due to a reduction in the blood supply to individual cells as the tumour enlarges. There is a tendency towards progressive hypoxia and partial tumour necrosis with increasing tumour size.

## Heterogeneity

Most cancers arise from one mutation in a single cell and so represent monoclonal proliferation, although further mutations are inevitable as the tumour grows. There are approximately $10^9$ cells within one cubic centimetre of tissue and most cancers are substantially larger than this when first detected. Thus most cancers are to some extent heterogeneous and this tendency towards heterogeneity increases as the tumour grows. Manifestations of heterogeneity include variations in cellular appearance, hormone receptor concentrations, and variations in the response to treatment in different metastases. The heterogeneity of cancer is thus a substantial block to successful treatment. Radiotherapy, hormone therapy and cytotoxic chemotherapy often fail because of the presence of a small number of cells which are resistant to attack. This is also likely to be a substantial problem in treatments using monoclonal antibodies.

## Invasion

The hallmark of malignant tumours is their ability to invade locally and to spread to distant sites. Local invasion is often much more extensive than is apparent macroscopically, accounting for the frequency of local recurrence following macroscopically adequate surgery. Malignant tumours do not form capsules, although the compression of surrounding tissues may occasionally create a false capsule. This is quite common in soft-tissue sarcomas, for example, for which mere 'shelling out' will almost always fail to remove all the malignant cells.

## Metastasis

Metastatic spread is a complicated process which occurs more frequently with undifferentiated, rapidly growing tumours.

Only a very small proportion of shed cells are capable of eventual development into overt distant tumours. For successful haematogenous spread, cells have to breach the vascular basement membrane within the primary tumour, survive transport in the blood stream, breach the basement membrane in a target organ and then proliferate in a foreign micro-environment, the characteristics of this micro-environment being crucial. The distribution of blood-borne metastases does not closely reflect the blood flow to different sites. Some primary carcinomas may remain undetectable even in the presence of enormous blood-borne or lymphatic metastases. Conversely, axillary lymphadenopathy, for example, does not become clinically apparent in patients with breast carcinoma with the frequency that might be expected from the known incidence of histological involvement.

The principal routes of metastatic spread are via blood and lymphatic vessels, although haematogenous spread does not necessarily imply dissemination throughout the blood stream. Only lung tumours have direct access to the arterial system; for other tumours arterial spread can occur only after shed cells have successfully negotiated the lungs or have established lung metastases. Spread via the paravertebral venous plexus probably accounts for the centripetal distribution of bone metastases from breast and prostate carcinomas.

Trans-coelomic spread occurs with a variety of tumours and is a particularly well recognised feature of ovarian carcinomas. Perineural spread is a form of local infiltration but can occasionally occur over several centimetres and is particularly recognised in malignant head and neck tumours. Some CNS tumours have a particular tendency to spread via the cerebro-spinal fluid. Dissemination via soft tissue planes is a feature of soft tissue sarcomas.

There is often a correlation between different facets of a tumour's aggressiveness. Larger, primary tumours are usually associated with a higher incidence of metastases. Whilst this may reflect a longer time during which metastasis could have occurred, it is often more likely to reflect an inherent potential for more malignant behaviour. Similarly, lymphatic spread may sometimes be indicative of an aggressive potential associated with a high risk of haematogenous spread. For such tumours treatment directed to the regional lymph nodes may have a low chance of influencing survival.

## Biochemistry

The cachexia which is sometimes seen with small malignant tumours is almost certainly due to tumour production of substances, largely unidentified, which interfere with normal metabolism. A large number of physiologically active agents secreted by tumours have been identified. These include amines, growth factors, polypeptide hormones and prostaglandins, some of which are responsible for well recognised 'paramalignant' phenomena including hypercalcaemia, inappropriate ADH secretion and gynaecomastia. The biochemical potential of malignant cells is crucial in determining a tumour's ability to infiltrate and metastasise. For example, the production of a specific collagenase confers an ability to penetrate vascular basement membranes, and the development of bone metastases *in vivo* is correlated to the ability of tissue from the primary tumour to cause osteolysis *in vitro*. The establishment of bone metastases depends on the production of locally active chemicals which cause initial osteolysis thus creating a space for invasion by the malignant cells.

## Immunology

Cellular and humoral responses to the presence of cancer are very well documented, but it has yet to be established whether such responses are beneficial. Many tumour 'antigens' have been identified but the use of the word 'antigen' is slightly misleading since it refers only to the method of immunological detection in the laboratory, not to the ability to evoke a useful, immunological response in the human host.

Congenital or acquired immune deficiency causes an increased risk of malignancy, but the increased risk is in specific malignancies, particularly those of components of the immune system, rather than reflecting the usual distribution of different cancers in the general population. Similarly, spontaneous regression, a very rare event, has a predilection for certain relatively uncommon malignancies such as neuroblastoma, lymphoma, choriocarcinoma, melanoma and renal carcinoma. Such observations certainly do not preclude the occurrence of useful immunological responses to malignant tumours, but they are not easily reconciled with the hypothesis that effective immunosurveillance eliminates the majority of cancers at an early stage. Much endeavour has gone into the study of tumour immunology and into therapeutic attempts to stimulate or augment immunological responses. Sadly there has been little clinical benefit so far, although it seems likely that useful advances will be made in this area. One interesting development has been the demonstration of tumour regression in some patients treated with preparations derived from lymphocytes infiltrating their own tumour. It is possible to promote the multiplication of these lymphocytes *in vitro* using a growth factor, interleukin-2, and then to re-infuse them. Responses have been seen in a few patients with melanoma and renal and lung carcinoma treated with tumour-infiltrating lymphocytes together with interleukin-2. The mechanism is uncertain, but it seems likely that the responses are mediated not through direct lysis by the infused lymphocytes, but through a stimulatory effect on endogenous cell-mediated responses.

## NOTES

# NOTES

# CHAPTER 2

# Treatment Intent

Much harm can be done, and valuable resources wasted, when the aim of medical intervention is not clarified at the outset. There are only two justifications for proceeding with anti-cancer treatments and these are the possibility of prolonging life and the possibility of relieving symptoms.

## Prolonging Life

Most anti-cancer treatment with surgery, radiotherapy or drugs, given with the principal intent of prolonging life, is given with the intent to cure. Approximately 40 per cent of all cancer patients in the western world are now cured, when 'cure' means death from something else, but only about 25 per cent are cured when patients with skin cancer are excluded. The possibility of cure should be carefully considered in the initial management of all cancer patients, even though it will often be immediately apparent that this is not feasible. The most common reasons for this are either the advanced state of the primary tumour or the presence of metastases.

To stand any chance of success, treatment given with the intent of cure must be given with the aim of complete tumour extirpation. The term 'radical' is often applied to such treatment, literally meaning removal by the roots [L. radix, a root]. Radical treatment with surgery, radiotherapy or chemotherapy often causes considerable morbidity but this is usually considered justifiable because of the magnitude of the potential benefit. It should not be forgotten, however, that to 'cure' is merely to postpone the inevitable, thereby allowing the patient to die eventually from something else. Attempts to cure theoretically curable patients may not always be thought justifiable after consideration of the actual chance of complete eradication of tumour, the age and general condition of the patient and the toxicity of treatment. Nevertheless, radical treatments may often be justifiably given when there is only a very remote chance of cure (for example rather aggressive cytotoxic chemotherapy for some patients with moderately advanced ovarian carcinoma or apparently localised small cell lung cancer) because the majority of those who will not be cured stand a reasonable chance of having their lives substantially prolonged by many months, or even a few years. Many other patients treated with methods with substantially higher chances of cure (for example surgery for patients with colorectal carcinoma or radiotherapy for those with advanced carcinomas of the cervix) will die of their disease a few years after treatment, but will undoubtedly have had their lives substantially prolonged by it.

The true extent of many tumours is often established only at operation and surgical exploration is often justifiably embarked upon in the hope that a radical procedure will be feasible. Even when it becomes apparent that cure is not possible many patients may benefit from palliative procedures, such as local excision, despite the presence of obvious metastases, or a by-pass procedure where there is an irresectable primary growth, in the belief that there is a reasonable chance of at least improving the quality of life.

# Relieving Symptoms

Treatment given with the principal aim of relieving symptoms is described as 'palliative', literally meaning a cloaking or covering of the manifestations of the disease [L. pallium, a cloak]. Since virtually all patients who are offered only palliative treatment are incurable it is usually considered desirable to minimise the aggressiveness of treatment, and thereby its toxicity, as far as possible. Dosages of palliative radiotherapy are, therefore, often less than half of those used in radical treatment. There is little point, however, in giving extremely well-tolerated treatment if it stands only a remote chance of achieving any palliative benefit. There is good evidence that some rather more aggressive palliative treatments result in a greater improvement in quality of life overall than other treatments which may be better tolerated. There is, however, no point in replacing the symptoms of the disease by different, but equal or more severe, symptoms from treatment. It is impossible to predict accurately the adverse effects of treatment for any individual patient. There will always be some patients who will react surprisingly badly and the relative chances of advantage and disadvantage should always be weighed up by an experienced clinician before the patient is offered palliative treatment. Disadvantages may include not only the side effects of treatment, but also the social disruption caused by travel to and from hospital or admission to the ward, although some patients seem to thrive on this.

There must always be a good reason for offering any palliative treatment. It is rarely justified in the absence of troublesome symptoms. However, quite a common problem arises when a patient, who has no troublesome symptoms, knows the diagnosis and expects treatment, or has been led to expect it. Sometimes a frank discussion and explanation that treatment will be of no benefit, or is likely to do more harm than good, will resolve the situation, but for a small number of patients it may be kinder to treat, liberally interpreting their anxiety about not being treated as a symptom; such clinical decision-making requires considerable sensitivity. Some patients have visible or palpable tumours that are causing no problems other than anxiety and again this may justify treatment. Occasionally, palliative treatment may be justified as a prophylactic measure, for example radiotherapy to a tumour which threatens to fungate, or to the mediastinum of a symptomless patient who has clinical signs of early superior vena caval obstruction.

Surgery, radiotherapy and anti-cancer drugs may all be used to palliate symptoms, but there are many patients for whom the best option is none of these because the symptoms are more likely to be relieved by other treatments such as analgesics. Some palliative treatments undoubtedly prolong the lives of those patients who respond to them, and occasionally they are given with prolongation of life as one of the main aims (for example cytotoxic chemotherapy for multiple myeloma) but most have little influence on survival. For the

great majority of patients treated palliatively any prolongation of life (which is often difficult to demonstrate convincing-
ly) is but a welcome addition to the relief of symptoms which is
the justification for treatment. It must never be forgotten that
some patients have their lives shortened by treatment given
with palliative intent.

## Investigations

When a patient is assessed initially as being eligible for
potentially curative treatment it is appropriate to arrange
any investigation which stands a reasonable chance of demonstrating incurability. Sometimes incurability is demonstrated by defining the extent of the primary tumour more
accurately but, more commonly, it is demonstrated by establishing the existence of metastatic spread. Such investigations should be arranged after consideration of the natural
history of the tumour concerned: a chest X-ray is justifiable in
almost all cancer patients other than those with non-melanomatous skin cancer, but investigations which stand very little
chance of altering management may sometimes only delay
effective treatment. Sometimes (as in Hodgkin's disease)
investigations are performed to define the extent of disease so
that the most suitable modality for potentially curative treatment can be used.

There is usually little need for much investigation prior to
palliative treatment since the requirement for treatment is
predominantly determined by symptoms. Some investigations may be justifiably ordered with the aim of reducing the
chance of iatrogenic morbidity, for example the testing of
renal function and estimation of full blood counts in patients
being considered for cytotoxic chemotherapy. X-rays are
often necessary to assist in the accurate localisation of
radiotherapy fields but, as in all routine clinical practice, no
investigation should be ordered unless it is likely to influence
management.

## Therapeutic ratio

This concept is the ratio of the effect of treatment against the
cancer over the adverse effects of treatment against the host.

Treatments that have a high therapeutic ratio are highly effective in dealing with the tumour whilst causing only slight morbidity. Where clinical experience indicates that a given treatment for a given condition usually has a high therapeutic ratio it may be justifiable to recommend it, whether the aim is cure or palliation. If, however, the therapeutic ratio is generally low, the treatment may be used where there is a chance of cure, but its use in palliation is difficult to justify.

## Deciding between management options

Consideration of the therapeutic ratios of the various treatment modalities forms a logical basis for decision-making. There is generally less scope for variation in radical treatment than there is with palliative treatment, because of well-established differences in the success rate with different approaches; no-one will attempt to eradicate a colonic carcinoma without surgery, or leukaemia without chemotherapy. Where a tumour appears to be truly localised local treatment with surgery or radiotherapy is usually the chosen option, not only because they are local treatments but also because drugs alone are unable to eradicate most solid tumours. Some tumours, for example breast cancer, are known to have a very high metastatic potential despite appearing to be localised on presentation. They are also known to be moderately sensitive to certain drugs and for tumours such as these the administration of an adjuvant drug treatment in addition to local treatment with surgery and/or radiotherapy has been shown to prolong survival for some patients.

Dilemmas are far more common when considering palliative rather than radical management. For these patients treatment is palliative only because of the lack of curative potential of any of the available modalities. It is often difficult to decide whether to recommend local radiotherapy or anti-cancer drug treatment or other methods of symptom control. Although in practice there may be several possible options, it is often reasonable and helpful to introduce one anti-cancer treatment at a time, to enable better assessment of the efficacy of individual treatments. Above all it is important never to forget the place for purely symptomatic measures in addition to whatever oncological treatments may be deemed appropriate.

Decision-making in palliative care is frequently difficult and often calls for considerable experience and sensitivity. It can sometimes be made easier by careful and systematic consideration of the following points:

1  The patient's general physical and mental state, and major concerns.
2  Whether the symptoms are widespread or localised.
3  The likely therapeutic ratios of different options.
4  The social disruption likely to be caused by different options.
5  Whether or not there is a reasonable chance that systemic treatment will reduce the requirement for further local treatment to other areas.
6  Whether or not there is a reasonable chance that one of the options will significantly prolong life of reasonable quality.

**NOTES**

# NOTES

# CHAPTER 3

# Comprehensive Care

As far as the patient's cancer is concerned, it is important to consider the appropriateness of *local*, *regional* and *systemic* treatment. For many patients one or more of these will be irrelevant but, in busy clinical practice, it is quite easy for potentially beneficial additional treatment, or alterations in treatment, to go by default. Examples include the possibilities that local palliative radiotherapy for bone pain might be beneficial for a patient with metastatic carcinoma of prostate undergoing orchidectomy, that whole pelvic radiotherapy might be advisable after surgery for a cervical carcinoma which involved lymphatics, and that a change in systemic hormonal medication or a switch to cytotoxic chemotherapy might be appropriate for a patient with metastatic breast carcinoma requiring palliative radiotherapy.

Good management of cancer patients involves substantially more than the diagnosis and treatment of the malignancy. Doctors should treat the whole patient rather than just the tumours; much harm can be done if the whole patient is not considered first and foremost. The following aspects of care should always be considered:

1 Symptom control
2 Attention to treatment toxicity
3 General medical care
4 Communication
5 Psychological support
6 Nursing, social and other paramedical support.

## 1 Symptom control

It is unfortunately still common for cancer patients to be receiving appropriate treatment for their tumour, but inadequate symptom control, particularly in the case of pain relief. Inadequate symptom control results not only in unnecessary physical suffering, but can also substantially impair morale and the ability to tolerate treatment.

## 2 Attention to treatment toxicity

Treatment with radiotherapy and cytotoxic chemotherapy is often prolonged and can cause severe and even life-threatening toxicity which may become manifest during treatment or after its completion. This is particularly the case with treatments given with curative intent. Early detection of potentially serious toxicity usually allows appropriate intervention with specific remedies, or temporary cessation of treatment before more serious sequelae supervene. Good management of treatment toxicity offers the best chance of satisfactorily completing the initially planned treatment, and can thus materially influence the chance of cure.

Prophylaxis is sometimes effective in reducing the morbidity from treatment. Examples include: the use of heparin prior to major surgery, the starting of anti-emetics on the day before cytotoxic chemotherapy, the avoidance of mucosal irritants (especially smoking) in patients receiving radiotherapy for head and neck cancer, the avoidance of urate nephropathy with allopurinol prior to cytotoxic chemotherapy for leukaemia or lymphoma and the attempted prevention of herpes infections with acyclovir in patients receiving highly immunosuppressive treatments.

## 3 General medical care

Cancer patients are often prone to general medical problems by virtue of their disease or its treatment, for example susceptibility to infections and hypercalcaemia, but many cancer patients are elderly and suffer from other illnesses totally unrelated to their malignancy. It must never be automatically assumed that an unexplained decline in general condition is due to uncontrollable neoplasia. This is a particularly dangerous assumption in patients otherwise thought to have potentially curable cancer.

For many cancer patients there may be entirely valid reasons for a 'do not resuscitate' instruction, but it is very dangerous to exclude any cancer patient from cardiopulmonary resuscitation without careful consideration. Successful resuscitation can result in some patients with advanced and incurable disease living many months or even years with good quality of life.

## 4 Communication

Ideally the patient should be given the opportunity to ask questions, voice concerns and say how he or she feels physically and psychologically, in a relaxed unhurried atmosphere. Pressure on time and resources often substantially interferes with this ideal, but at the very least every new patient should be invited to ask questions.

It is almost always helpful to ask patients what they already understand about their condition and what they have been told. Patients will often say at first they have been told 'nothing at all' but will then go on to say they know they have or have had cancer, what has been done so far and what further treatment they have been led to expect. Others will continue to profess ignorance about their condition when there is indisputable evidence that they have been told.

Every patient has an absolute right to know their own diagnosis and the likely prognosis, if they really wish to know the truth. Most patients who really want to know the exact situation will make their feelings fairly clear. The great majority of cancer patients either know or very strongly suspect the diagnosis. However, many will not ask because they do not wish this to be made explicit. This may be because they feel they could not cope and/or because their hope is tethered to the belief that they may not have cancer. Many of those who do ask want to be told only that they do not have cancer or will be cured of it. This too is usually apparent, but appropriate communication calls for considerable sensitivity, not only to the spoken word but to non-verbal cues such as facial expression and general bearing.

The views of relatives concerning communication with the patient should be taken seriously, even though the doctor's duty is entirely to the patient. By far the most important, and sometimes the overriding, factor should be the doctor's considered assessment of how much the patient should be told. Many relatives express the view that they feel the patient could not cope with being told the truth whilst in fact the patient knows, or very strongly suspects, what that truth is. Every patient and social situation is however different and whilst a 'conspiracy of silence' between the patient and relatives can substantially impair the quality of life at home for some, for others this may be the most appropriate adjustment to the situation.

There is never any justification for lying to a patient. This is a fundamental denial of their autonomy as well as posing all sorts of practical problems with the subsequent risk of loss of faith. However there is often every justification for being economical with the truth, releasing it sometimes hardly at all, sometimes very gradually and often never completely, in accordance with a sensitive assessment of how much the patient really wants to know. It is usually possible to present information in an optimistic light without telling an untruth. It is rarely justifiable to extinguish all hope, but for some patients all their hope is for the next world and can never be extinguished.

In theory a doctor should not normally divulge information about a patient to anyone without the patient's consent, although in practice it is often permissible, proper and helpful to impart information concerning the diagnosis and prognosis to the next-of-kin. Information given to the patient may be packaged appropriately in an optimistic light, whilst the next-of-kin should be told the situation exactly as the doctor sees it. Passing on this information is often of considerable help to the patient in several ways.

It must not be forgotten that the doctor primarily responsible for a patient's care is their general practitioner. Good communication with the GP is essential as it will often enable him to do the very best for the patient at home. He should be told not only the diagnosis and treatment given or planned, but any anticipated further developments including treatment-related morbidity, the likely prognosis, plans for hospital follow-up, medication on discharge and, very importantly, what the patient and next-of-kin have been told.

## 5  Psychological support

As many as 25 per cent of cancer patients suffer from clinic-ally-significant depression and anxiety and, for certain groups of patients, e.g. those receiving prolonged adjuvant cytotoxic chemotherapy, the incidence is somewhat higher. Psychological morbidity is not only unpleasant in itself but can seriously impair the ability of a patient to cope with treatment, sometimes resulting in its premature termination. Counselling and psychotropic drugs are often helpful for these conditions which are usually considerably underdiagnosed.

## 6  Nursing, social and other paramedical support

This is often rather more important than anything the doctor can do himself and embraces a wide spectrum of care. In hospital it may include breast, stoma and incontinence nursing services, medical social work services, and occupational and speech therapy. In the community it may include relatives and friends, hospice and district nursing services, home helps, meals on wheels, charitable organisations and self-help groups.

Consideration of all possible community support is particularly relevant for the frail, the elderly, and those who are incurable. Medical social workers play a crucial rôle in assessing requirements and mobilising appropriate support, and also in arranging financial help where necessary. Such measures will often make a substantial impact on the quality of life for patients and may enable them to stay in their own homes.

# NOTES

# CHAPTER 4

# Admission Practice

An especially comprehensive history and clinical examination on admission to the ward is not always appropriate or necessary, particularly for those patients who have already been diagnosed and for those who are being repeatedly readmitted. There are usually constraints on time and it is important that the time spent by a doctor with a patient newly arrived on the ward is used most effectively. It is also important that resources are not wasted by arranging for unnecessary investigations.

## History-taking

Care should be taken to elicit all of the patient's current symptoms. Many patients are inclined to think, wrongly, that some symptoms are not relevant. The development of new, or the disappearance of old, symptoms is often a crucial factor leading to changes in management. If a patient says that he or she can feel a lump this should always be taken very seriously, even if it appears to be impalpable.

The social history is also important, particularly such aspects as the support services available at home (lay and professional, physical and psychological), the proximity and helpfulness of relatives, friends and neighbours, and the structural suitability of the patients' home when they are significantly incapacitated.

A relatively detailed occupational history is important on one occasion. Some tumours, particularly bladder cancer and

mesothelioma, are known to be caused by industrial carci-
nogens and compensation may be available. The causative
exposure may have taken place many years previously.

Patients should usually be asked if they understand what is
the matter with them and given the rationale for their clinical
management. They should then be given the opportunity to
ask questions and to voice any worries.

# Examination

The possibility that this will usefully influence or alter management should always be borne in mind.

## The primary tumour

It is important to palpate tumours and not just rely on a visual
examination. Some tumours are often more extensive than
they appear initially. This should not be forgotten when
examining tumours within the mouth and (if palpation is
possible) the oropharynx. Primary tumours and lymphadenopathy should be tested for mobility and tethering to surrounding structures. Deep tethering of breast tumours is detectable
by a reduction in mobility when the patient's ipselateral hand
is pressed firmly inwards on the waist. The appearance and
temperature of the overlying skin should be noted. In fungating tumours a characteristic unpleasant smell may indicate a
treatable superadded anaerobic infection.

There is often quite marked observer variation in assessment of tumour size and, whenever possible, sequential
measurements should be performed by the same observer
using the same technique. The size of lumps deep to the skin is
best detected by light palpation in a vertical plane; the position of the underlying tumour margins can then be defined on
the surface using a skin marker. Compression of the tumour
will lead to a falsely high estimate of size since the palpable
lump will include a component of overlying normal tissue.

## Lymphadenopathy

Patients who have been thought suitable for radical local treatment should be examined with the particular aim of detecting any palpable or visible metastases. The relevant regional lymph node areas should always be palpated carefully and, in particular, both supraclavicular fossae should be thoroughly examined in all patients with visceral and breast carcinomas. Lymphatic spread from intra-abdominal or pelvic tumours is usually to the left supraclavicular fossa but can be to the right. Supraclavicular lymphadenopathy is often situated very deeply and medially and can sometimes be detected only in either the upright or the supine position. The supraclavicular fossae should be examined both from behind and from the front. Some patients with breast carcinoma develop infraclavicular lymphadenopathy but this region is often not palpated. The axilla is best examined with the patient's ipselateral arm relaxed and resting on the examining forearm of the doctor; bimanual palpation may be helpful. In cases of doubt an enlarged axillary lymph node can usually be distinguished from other structures, when the examining fingers are rolled over it, by being clearly palpable as a prominent lump in both of two planes at right-angles. Internal mammary lymphadenopathy occasionally becomes clinically apparent in breast cancer patients, usually causing an ill-defined bulge in the region of the upper costo-chondral junctions. Mediastinal and supraclavicular lymphadenopathy may cause a hoarse voice from recurrent laryngeal nerve palsy, particularly in lung cancer patients. Epitrochlear lymphadenopathy may occur from tumours on the hands or forearms, and in patients with lymphomas. Most patients should have their legs examined – para-aortic lymphadenopathy may cause backache and bilateral leg oedema, whilst pelvic lymphadenopathy is more likely to cause unilateral leg swelling.

It is very important to detect neck lymphadenopathy in patients with head and neck cancer. The neck should be palpated bilaterally from behind. A tortuous carotid artery is occasionally mistaken for lymphadenopathy, but of course it is pulsatile. The hyoid bone is also mistaken for lymphadenopathy but the lumpiness is symmetrically bilateral and moves on one side when pressure is applied on the other. Crepitus should normally be elicited when the larynx is pressed backwards and moved from side to side over the cervical vertebrae. Loss of crepitus may indicate pre-vertebral primary tumour extension or lymphadenopathy.

## Bone metastases

Metastatic bone involvement is often tender to light percussion with the medial side of the examiner's fist; this should be tested for gently. Local tenderness to percussion however does not always indicate underlying pathology; tenderness, like pain, can occasionally be referred.

## Hepatomegaly

Malignant hepatomegaly is quite often not palpable but right hypochondrial tenderness is frequently an indication of its presence.

## Serious complications

Any inspiratory stridor in patients with tumours involving the upper respiratory tract must be detected. Only a slight additional narrowing in an already compromised airway may cause minimal stridor to become pronounced, with severe respiratory difficulty.

Spinal cord or cauda equina compression must be detected at as an early a stage as possible. A thorough neurological examination should be performed in any patient who complains of leg weakness or numbness, or loss of sphincter control. In particular, such patients should be examined for the presence of a sensory level by light pin-prick testing from the legs upwards. It should be remembered that there is a discrepancy between dermatomes and the vertebral level of a lesion. As a rough rule there is a discrepancy of one in the cervical spine, two in the thoracic spine and three in the lumbar spine; for example a sensory level at T8 dermatome may be caused by a lesion in the 6th thoracic vertebra. Such patients often exhibit tenderness to light percussion over the relevant vertebra if it is the site of metastatic disease, but some patients will have neurological compression by metastatic tumour without involvement of the adjacent bone. It is also important to detect superior vena caval obstruction as soon as possible. A slight suggestion of facial swelling or plethora is often the first indication. The external jugular veins show no variation in distension with the cardiac cycle and there is quite often a slight vascular flare visible just beneath the breasts.

A very thorough examination should be performed on immunocompromised patients who are febrile. This will include examination of the skin for rash or source of infection, mouth and oropharynx, ears, perineum (but not necessarily rectum for fear of causing or exacerbating bacteraemia), fundi and testing for meningism.

Patients who have evidence of right heart failure or breathlessness not explained in other ways may have a pericardial effusion. This is seen most commonly with carcinomas of the breast and bronchus. There will usually be detectable pulsus 'paradoxus' (often best palpated at the femoral arteries), a weak or absent apex beat and often a pericardial rub.

## Unknown primaries

Some patients present with metastatic tumours from an unknown primary site. If the metastatic disease is lymphadenopathy a thorough search should be made of the area drained by the involved nodes whenever this is clinically accessible. Patients with metastatic tumour should be examined especially with the aim of discovering a primary site which might indicate the possibility of a relatively treatable neoplasm. In particular the breasts (both males and females) should be palpated systematically and carefully with the flat of the combined middle three fingers and with the patient supine; the axillae and supraclavicular fossae should also be palpated. The thyroid and prostate should be palpated and the pelvis examined for rectal or uterine carcinoma, and particularly for the presence of an adnexal (ovarian) mass. The testes should be examined and the presence of any gynaecomastia noted. This is often just a small subareolar pad which may be tender and unilateral.

# Investigations

Investigations should be arranged only if they stand a chance of usefully influencing clinical management. Investigations of purely academic interest should be requested only with the patient's informed consent. In the care of patients with known or suspected cancer the main justifications for investigations are as follows:

1  To establish the diagnosis
2  To define the extent of the disease
3  To discover the cause for symptoms
4  To assess the suitability for proposed treatment
5  To assess the response to treatment.

## Establishing the diagnosis

The crucial investigation is obtaining tissue for cytological or histological examination. Time and resources are often wasted, and avoidable patient discomfort caused, by investigations which stand no chance of getting to the crux of the problem.

Patients who present with metastatic carcinoma from an unknown primary should not always be routinely investigated to discover the primary site. It may benefit them to discover an origin in certain organs since some carcinomas stand a greater chance of usefully responding to relatively non-toxic systemic treatment, for example carcinomas of breast, prostate, ovary and thyroid. There is, however, no justification for submitting such patients to barium studies, intravenous urography or CT scans when relevant symptoms are absent. Patients who present with neck lymphadenopathy other than purely in the supraclavicular fossa should have a thorough ENT examination (and if necessary blind biopsies of the nasopharynx) since surgery or radiotherapy to the lymphadenopathy and primary site can sometimes be curative.

## Defining the extent of disease

This is justified only if the findings stand a reasonable chance of usefully influencing management, for example by determining the extent of a localised tumour prior to radical surgery or radiotherapy, or by establishing the presence of incurable metastases, thereby rendering radical local treatment unnecessary. It is also justified for determining whether radical treatment should be systemic (cytotoxic chemotherapy) or local (radiotherapy) in patients who present with clinically localised Hodgkin's disease or non-Hodgkin's lymphoma.

Patients with newly diagnosed and clinically localised breast carcinoma should be routinely tested for abnormal liver and bone enzymes but, in the absence of any symptoms suggestive of bone metastases, routine isotope bone scans are of little value. A routine chest X-ray is a justifiable investigation in the majority of patients presenting with apparently localised malignancy, other than non-melanomatous skin cancer.

## Discovering the cause for symptoms

Again, thought should be given to whether discovery of the cause will benefit the patient. Although this is usually far more relevant to palliative care, the discovery of possibly curable causes for symptoms in potentially curable patients is particularly important, for example pyrexia in immunocompromised patients with leukaemia or lymphoma.

Radiological investigations which establish metastatic disease as a cause for bone pain, lymphangitis carcinomatosa as a cause for dyspnoea and spinal cord compression as a cause for leg weakness, and laboratory investigations which establish anaemia as a cause for weakness and hypercalcaemia as a cause of nausea and thirst are all examples of tests which may lead to highly beneficial treatment for troublesome symptoms. As a general rule the simpler investigations should be done first, again only if they stand a reasonable chance of establishing the cause of the problem. X-rays usually show only metastatic bone disease when there is substantial involvement. Isotope bone scans are considerably more sensitive but these, too, are not foolproof. Patients with osteolysis from myeloma may have very little osteoblastic response and a normal serum alkaline phosphatase and isotope bone scan. X-rays can be arranged more quickly than isotope scans, can sometimes better localise disease prior to local radiotherapy, and can demonstrate pathological fractures, but isotope scans may still be a reasonable first option, particularly in patients with milder and less localised pain.

## Assessing suitability for proposed treatment

Important examples of investigations which are performed principally to assess whether or not the proposed treatment is likely to be tolerated are the biochemical and haematological investigations performed prior to cytotoxic chemotherapy. Impaired renal or liver function may substantially influence drug metabolism or excretion, with potentially serious consequences, and treatment with some nephrotoxic drugs, for example cisplatinum, demands repeated testing of renal function. Full blood counts must be performed immediately prior to every course of cytotoxic chemotherapy: proceeding with further treatment in the face of leucopenia or thrombocytopenia can be life-threatening. Another important example is the detection of anaemia prior to surgery or radical radiotherapy. Radiotherapy is likely to be less effective in the presence of anaemia since hypoxia causes radioresistance. Patients receiving radical radiotherapy should therefore be transfused if necessary.

Lung function tests are essential prior to pulmonary lobectomy or pneumonectomy. Patients with lung cancer often have obstructive airways disease: there is no point in radical removal of a tumour if there is not likely to be enough lung tissue remaining to sustain life of any quality.

## Assessing response to treatment

This is chiefly applicable to drug treatment which, in contrast to surgery and radiotherapy, can be relatively prolonged. When it is being given for overt disease (not adjuvantly), it is usually possible to assess the efficacy of treatment before it is completed. It is pointless to continue with treatment if the tumour continues to progress. In particular there is no justification for proceeding with a further pulse of cytotoxic chemotherapy, with its accompanying toxicity, if it can be established that it is ineffective. Visible or palpable lesions must therefore be measured every time.

There may be little justification in arranging investigations prior to every pulse of treatment if there has been obvious clinical improvement, although radiological and biochemical investigations (for example acid phosphatase in prostate carcinoma patients) are certainly justified if there is a possibility of tumour progression on clinical grounds and if the findings stand a reasonable chance of usefully influencing management. In the radical chemotherapy of testicular germ cell tumours and choriocarcinoma the serum concentration of tumour markers ($\beta$-HCG and/or $\alpha$-fetoprotein) should be very closely monitored.

There is no point in assessing response to treatment when the findings are unlikely to influence management usefully. For example, in prostate carcinoma, routine follow-up isotope bone scans after local radical treatment or orchidectomy for metastases are not necessary in the absence of new symptoms.

# Post-mortem Examinations

The great majority of cancer patients already have a tissue diagnosis prior to death, and the great majority of those with uncontrolled tumour die either directly, or indirectly, as a result of it. Although post-mortem examinations quite often demonstrate more extensive disease than had been previously recognised, they give a low yield of useful new information when carried out routinely, and are expensive. They should however be seriously considered in cases of sudden death or rapid unexpected decline. Requests for post-mortem examination should ideally be written by, or made after consultation with, the clinician primarily or predominantly responsible for the patient's management. Important information may otherwise not be given to the pathologist and this can compromise the usefulness of the investigation.

# NOTES

# CHAPTER 5

# Surgery

Most cancer patients are initially referred to surgeons, and the cytological or histological confirmation of malignancy established by some sort of surgical technique, from a fine needle aspirate to a laparotomy. Achieving a tissue diagnosis may sometimes call for considerable technical expertise, for example when obtaining biopsies from a small breast abnormality demonstrated on a screening mammogram, or from an area of osteolytic vertebra. The extent of the malignancy may also be established at surgery, and sometimes surgery may be undertaken specifically for this purpose. Examples of this include axillary lymph node sampling for patients with breast carcinoma, and staging laparotomy in patients with Hodgkin's disease.

## Surgery with Curative Intent

Surgery cures more patients of cancer than do both radiotherapy and cytotoxic chemotherapy together. Although surgery inevitably fails to cure when there is widespread disease, or when local excision is incomplete, the surest way of eradicating any truly localised tumour is, where possible, to excise it together with an adequate margin of normal tissue.

Attempts to remove technically operable tumours are not always in the patient's best interest however, particularly in the presence of advanced age or poor general health. The continuation of planned radical surgery despite the intra-operative discovery of lymphatic or haematogenous spread is also of debatable value.

Most cancer surgery is conducted as a 'cold' procedure. However, some patients present with symptoms such as perforation, haemorrhage or obstruction and these require emergency surgery. The results of emergency surgery are often relatively poor, usually reflecting the advanced stage of the tumours and often the patients' poor general condition.

## Conservative surgery

There has been a trend in recent decades towards less radical surgery for some tumours. This has been particularly applicable to breast carcinoma, due principally to the realisation that for most patients extensive local or regional (lymph node) involvement is indicative of the presence of an aggressive tumour which has already formed occult distant metastases. These patients will therefore remain incurable by even very extensive local treatment.

Local control does however remain very important for many patients, whether or not there is more distant spread. For patients with breast carcinoma and soft tissue sarcomas it has been established that relatively conservative surgery is often adequate, provided that subsequent radiotherapy is given to eradicate any local residual microscopic tumour. The consequent improved cosmesis and function can have a major impact on the quality of life. More conservative surgery has also become feasible for certain patients with osteogenic sarcoma. New prosthetic bone replacement techniques have facilitated limb-sparing surgery where previously an amputation would have been the only option.

## Surgery for metastases

For some patients with extensive loco-regional disease surgery can still be curative, for example those with regional lymph node involvement at presentation, or subsequently, from carcinomas of the skin, head and neck and large bowel. There are also some long-term apparently-cured survivors after resection of involved axillary nodes for breast carcinoma. Surgery is usually the choice of treatment for mobile lymph node metastases after the primary treatment of carcinomas, and can be curative for a minority, especially for those with lymphadenopathy from squamous carcinomas of the skin or head and neck.

Resection of haematogenous metastases can also be followed by long-term survival and cure in selected patients, especially those with solitary or very few metastases from relatively indolent tumours. Examples include lung spread from osteosarcomas, teratomas, renal carcinomas and soft tissue sarcomas, and liver spread from colorectal carcinomas. The chance of success tends to be greater for those with a long interval between treatment to the primary growth and the development of metastases.

## Alternative modalities

For the majority of tumours treatable by surgery there is no alternative treatment modality worth considering. For some cancers however, for example those of the head and neck or cervix and skin, radiotherapy may be of comparable efficacy. It may therefore be the preferred initial treatment because, for example, it is not mutilating or is simpler. It may sometimes be apparent at surgery that the patient would benefit from subsequent radiotherapy and the surgeon may leave metal clips at the site of residual tumour which will be visible on X-rays taken for radiotherapy planning.

## Importance of expertise

As with other modalities, patients with certain tumours stand a clearly better chance of cure if they are operated on by surgeons with particular expertise. Rates of local recurrence and survival can vary considerably between different surgeons, and sometimes there seems to be no reason other than a variation in surgical technique. Sometimes it is necessary to combine surgical skills, for example, optimal management for some patients with advanced head and neck carcinoma may involve two surgeons from different sub-specialties (ENT and plastic surgery) operating together.

## Assessment of response

For some tumours, for example ovarian and gastro-intestinal carcinomas, there are advocates of surgery as a 'second-look' procedure, performed to detect any 'recurrent' tumour at an asymptomatic stage when further excision may stand a reasonable chance of success. As yet, however, there has been little evidence that this significantly improves the chance of cure.

## Transfusion

It is generally considered necessary for patients with haemoglobin concentrations <10 g/dl to be transfused prior to elective surgery, because of the increased anaesthetic risks associated with anaemia. However, there have been reports that blood transfusion is associated with a reduced chance of cure for some cancers, specifically gastro-intestinal and breast carcinomas, and it has also been suggested that transfusion may exert an adverse immunological influence. It has been reported that the increased risk is found in patients who have received whole blood rather than packed red cells. All this remains somewhat controversial, however, and it may be that the observed associations are due to patients with an inherently worse prognosis having an increased requirement for transfusion. Nevertheless, a strong case can be made for avoiding perioperative transfusion unless it is clearly necessary, and for giving red blood cells rather than whole blood.

# Palliative Surgery

The rôle of surgery as a palliative treatment is often not fully appreciated or adequately considered. There are many examples of surgical (or semi-surgical) palliative procedures:

Amputation of useless, fungating or painful limbs
Biliary drainage (endoscopic or percutaneous) for biliary obstruction
By-pass procedures for gastro-intestinal obstruction
Colostomy as a defunctioning procedure for bowel obstruction
Cryosurgery for exophytic and/or haemorrhagic tumour
Diathermy for exophytic and/or haemorrhagic tumour
Embolisation for painful hepatomegaly or haemorrhage

Excision of symptom-causing primary tumour in incurable disease

Excision of metastases (e.g. in lungs or brain – occasionally curative)

Flap repair after excision of chest wall involvement with breast carcinoma

Homan's operation for lymphoedema

Hypophysectomy for pain relief from advanced breast or prostate carcinoma

Internal fixation for pathological fracture (sometimes prophylactic)

Laminectomy for spinal cord or cauda equina compression

Laser destruction of exophytic tumour in oesophagus or upper airways

Mastectomy for locally advanced breast carcinoma

Nephrostomy for ureteric obstruction

Nerve or ganglion blocks, ablation or transection for pain

Oesophageal intubation (usually endoscopic) for dysphagia

Omental transposition for chest wall disease from breast carcinoma

Oophorectomy as endocrine ablation for advanced breast carcinoma

Orchidectomy for metastatic prostate carcinoma

Pericardial window for recurrent pericardial effusion

Peritoneo-caval subcutaneous shunt for intractable ascites

Pleurectomy for recurrent pleural effusion

Pleurodesis for recurrent pleural effusion

Tracheostomy for upper airways obstruction

Ventriculo-caval or -peritoneal shunt for obstructive hydrocephalus

It is essential that patients are selected carefully for palliative surgical procedures, particularly those that are more extensive. In general, palliative surgery is most likely to be justifiable for patients in relatively good general condition and for those with more indolent tumours and a reasonable life expectancy. Consideration should be given to the possibility that another modality, or no treatment, might be more appropriate. It can often be cruel to subject dying patients to surgery as opposed to conservative management. This may particularly apply to procedures involving colostomy or urinary diversion. The majority of terminally ill patients with neoplastic bowel obstruction can be successfully cared for medically, and nephrostomy for uraemia secondary to advanced pelvic tumour may merely serve to allow the patient to die rather more unpleasantly only a short while later.

## NOTES

# CHAPTER 6

# Radiotherapy

Although total body irradiation is occasionally given, both with radical and palliative intent, the great majority of treatments with radiotherapy are localised to one part of the body. A potential advantage of radiotherapy over surgery is that a considerably greater volume of tissue can usually be treated, but it must be recognised that the treated tumour cells are not inevitably eradicated; radiation-induced cell death can rarely be guaranteed. Both modalities suffer from the inevitability of failure to cure if there is tumour outside the volume of tissue treated.

## Radiobiology

Ionising radiation can damage the DNA within the cell nucleus and thus prevent mitosis. Some DNA radiation damage can be repaired, usually within 4–5 hours. A variable proportion of any individual radiation dose goes in causing repairable damage, the size of the proportion being larger the smaller the dose. Effective unrepaired radiation damage is usually made manifest by cell death as it attempts to undergo mitosis. This does not necessarily occur at the first mitosis after exposure to irradiation: sometimes a few cell cycles take place before radiation death.

### Radiation tumour damage

*Radiosensitivity* is a measure of the ability of a given radiation dose to eradicate a tumour completely. *Radiocurability* is a measure of the ability to deliver, with relative safety, a radiation dose that can destroy the tumour. *Radioresponsive-*

*ness* is the term used to describe the rate of shrinkage of a tumour after irradiation; it is indirectly related to radiosensitivity and does not necessarily imply radiocurability.

Some tumours, for example some skin basal cell carcinomas, are only slowly radioresponsive, but nevertheless in time (sometimes over several months) they may be completely eradicated by the treatment, i.e. they are highly radiocurable. In this particular example the dose required for cure is quite high and so these tumours are not regarded as being very radiosensitive, even though they are nearly always radiocurable. Other tumours, for example localised non-Hodgkin's lymphomas, often respond rapidly to irradiation (sometimes disappearing over a few days) and are therefore regarded as highly radioresponsive as well as radiosensitive and radiocurable. In general, tumours that look unchanged in size several weeks after starting a course of radiotherapy stand a poor chance of eventual eradication, although this does not mean that treatment failure is necessarily inevitable.

## Factors affecting radiation response

Because cell death usually becomes apparent at mitosis, the rate of shrinkage after effective irradiation will depend on the proportion of tumour cells within the mitotic cycle, and on the cell cycle time. It will also be influenced by the percentage of tumour cells that are not part of the malignant clone and the effectiveness of clearance of dead tumour cells and stromal cells from the tumour site; this may depend on the vascularity. Ultimate success or failure will depend on the impact of radiation on the tumour stem cell population.

Some stromal cells (e.g. fibroblasts) are relatively poorly radioresponsive whilst others (e.g. lymphocytes) are highly radioresponsive. Tumours with a high reactive lymphocytic component, for example Hodgkin's disease, may show a rapid initial reduction in size following treatment, which may not necessarily indicate tumour cell radiosensitivity. In contrast, the stromal fibrous tissue component sometimes extensively present in Hodgkin's disease, as well as in other tumours, may result in the persistence of a lump long after all malignant cells have been eradicated. Despite these possibilities, however, there is in general a fairly good correlation between the short- or medium-term clinical impression of a good response to treatment and long-term local control. Effective treatment for rapidly growing tumours will usually be apparent soon after starting treatment, whilst that for indolent tumours often results only in slow shrinkage. Any tumour that grows during or after radiotherapy stands virtually no chance of being eradicated by it.

Oxygen is very important to the process of DNA damage caused by the free radicals produced by ionising radiation, and less damage will be caused in the presence of hypoxia. It is believed that the presence of hypoxia within some tumours, partly as a result of inadequate vasculature, may be an important factor limiting their radiocurability.

Another reason for the failure of radiotherapy to eradicate some tumours is the continued replication of undamaged tumour cells during treatment. At the cellular level radiotherapy is very much a 'hit or miss' affair and a given dose of irradiation will tend to destroy an equal *proportion* of the total cell population, and not an equal number of cells, at each treatment. There is thus a tendency for the destruction of tumour cells to proceed exponentially. Successful treatment depends on either complete eradication of all clonogenic malignant cells, or eradication of all but a very small number, which may then be destroyed by host mechanisms. Continued replication of cells during treatment will increase the total number of targets to be destroyed by the prescribed radiation dose, and will thus diminish the chance of cure. This phenomenon may be particularly important because the continued replication of undamaged cells may actually be stimulated by their increased nutrition during treatment, as a result of the death of other cells previously drawing on the tumour vasculature.

## Radiation normal tissue damage

Every cancer could theoretically be eradicated by giving a high enough dose to an adequate volume of tissue, but such an approach would kill most patients. It is the damage to normal tissues which limits both the radiation dose and the volume of tissue treated.

## Degenerative change

Normal tissues vary in their radioresponsiveness and radiosensitivity. Rapidly proliferating tissues such as bone marrow, gut epithelium and skin are the first to show radiation damage. The lungs and gonads (particularly the latter, where fertility is affected in both sexes and hormonal synthesis affected in females only) are also very radiosensitive. For these tissues long-term radiosensitivity can also be marked: in particular gonadal radiation damage tends to be permanent after quite low doses. Although the bone marrow is exquisitely sensitive to low radiation doses adequate haemopoiesis is usually maintained by compensatory increased activity in non-irradiated marrow, and by the subsequent migration of marrow stem cells via the blood stream into areas that have been irradiated. Other tissues that are very radiosensitive in the long term include the lens and kidneys. Bone, muscle and connective tissues are relatively radioresistant in the adult, whilst the central nervous system and liver are intermediate. Bone growth is very susceptible to irradiation and this has important implications for paediatric radiotherapy.

Short-term normal tissue damage principally involves just an acute loss of cells. Long-term damage may also involve an effect on the endothelium of small blood vessels causing ischaemia or necrosis, and fibrosis. Normal cells, like malignant cells, can repair radiation damage. The ability to destroy tumours with irradiation without causing necrosis of the surrounding normal tissues depends on the balance between the repair potential in normal cells and the overall radiosensitivity of the malignant cells. The former is often the limiting factor, especially when large volumes of normal tissue are irradiated.

## Neoplastic change

The induction of overt cancer by radiotherapy is very rare. Since this occurs as a result of a mutation in a single cell it takes a long while for the tumour to become apparent. Usually radiation-induced leukaemia or lymphoma takes at least 5 years to become manifest, whilst other tumours take at least

10 years. One reason for its apparent rarity is therefore the death of many patients before a second malignancy could have been discovered. Another important reason is the lack of a linear relationship between dose and tumour induction. The incidence of tumour induction at first rises with increasing dose but then falls progressively within the dose range often used in clinical practice. This is thought to be due to radiation death in cells which have just undergone malignant transformation as a result of DNA damage. Radiation-induced malignancy is a somewhat more important factor in paediatric oncology, given the success of many treatments and the otherwise long life expectancy.

# Therapy

There are two main modes of delivery of radiotherapy, *teletherapy* and *brachytherapy*. Teletherapy involves the use of treatment machines to produce a beam or beams of radiation which enter the body from the outside. Brachytherapy involves the placing of the source of radiation within or very close to the tumour. Most teletherapy is given with electromagnetic irradiation produced by machines which generate X-rays or release gamma (γ) rays from radioisotopes. X-rays and γ-rays have identical physical properties and it is only their mode of production that is different. Brachytherapy is given using radioisotopes which release γ-rays or beta (β) particles (electrons). Radioisotopes may also be administered systemically or distributed within body cavities in solution or colloidal form.

## Radiation production

### Electromagnetic radiation

This embraces a vast spectrum, from radio-waves at one end (very low energy and frequency and very long wavelength) via infra-red, visible light and ultraviolet to X-rays and γ-rays at the other (very high energy and frequency and very short wavelength). X-rays and γ-rays have sufficient energy to cause ionisation, which is the removal of an electron from its atom or molecule. Ionisation is the basis of radiation damage to DNA. All electromagnetic irradiation obeys the inverse square law: the intensity is inversely proportional to the square of the distance from the source. This has important implications for both radiotherapy and for the protection of personnel from radiation (see below).

## X-rays

These are produced by accelerating electrons so that they hit a metal target at high energy. Some of their kinetic energy is then converted into electromagnetic radiation. The acceleration is either achieved by the application of a potential difference across a gap in a conventional X-ray tube, or if very high energy X-rays are required, by the use of radiowaves to carry the electrons down the wave guide of a linear accelerator. Any given machine will produce a spectrum of X-ray energies, the energy of the machine being defined by the maximum X-ray energy produced. The maximum energy of the rays in the diagnostic X-ray spectra is usually in the 50–150 kilo-electron-volt (keV) energy range. This is approximately the same energy as is used in *superficial* therapy rays for the treatment of skin tumours, although here the total amount of radiation delivered is infinitely greater. Diagnostic X-rays are usually produced for less than a second whilst superficial radiotherapy may be given over several minutes with the X-ray source much closer to the patient. The maximum energy of the *orthovoltage* or 'deep' therapeutic X-ray spectra is usually 250–300 keV, and these beams are used to treat tumours at a depth of a few centimetres. Linear accelerators produce much more deeply penetrating *megavoltage* beams with energies in the 4–25 million-electron-volt (meV) range.

## γ-rays

These are produced by the decay of a radioactive isotope. Isotopes decay continuously, although the rate of emission of radiation declines with time, according to the half-life of the isotope. The most commonly used isotopic alternative to X-ray production is $^{60}Co$, a radioisotope of cobalt. This has a half-life of 5 years and so the radiation source needs to be replaced every 3–4 years, otherwise treatments become very prolonged. The small source is sealed within the middle of a large lead unit which prevents the leakage of radiation when not in use. During treatment a small window is opened in the lead unit allowing the escape of γ-rays. $^{60}$Co produces mega-voltage γ-rays of a constant energy approximately equivalent to a 3 meV linear accelerator beam.

Radioactive caesium ($^{137}$Cs) is the most commonly used isotope for brachytherapy, particularly in the management of gynaecological malignancy. Other radioisotopes used for brachytherapy include iridium ($^{192}$Ir) and tantalum ($^{182}$Ta).

## β-rays or electrons

Some isotopes emit electrons (relatively low energy), which are also known as β-particles or -rays. These may be the only type of radiation emitted (e.g. from radioactive phosphorus [$^{32}$P]), or they may be emitted together with γ-rays (for example, from radioactive iodine [$^{131}$I] or radioactive gold [$^{98}$Au]). β-particles can only penetrate a few millimetres from the source of irradiation.

Many radiotherapy departments now have linear accelerators which can deliver high energy electron beams as well as X-rays. The electrons accelerated in the wave guide are released without hitting the tungsten-copper target. Most electron treatments are given using a single beam, the principle advantage of electron beams over X- or γ-rays being that they are more rapidly attenuated at depth. They are thus particularly useful in delivering a high dose to tumours at or near the surface whilst at the same time delivering a substantially lower dose to deeper normal structures. Their penetration is proportional to their energy and the beam energy chosen depends on the depth of tissue requiring treatment with a cancerocidal dose.

## Neutrons

Treatment with neutrons is still largely experimental. The principal theoretical advantage of treatment with high energy (fast) neutrons (usually produced in a cyclotron) is that they produce very dense ionisation which, compared with X- and γ-rays, results in less repair of DNA damage. The damage is also less dependent on the presence of oxygen and so the presence of hypoxia in a tumour is less likely to cause radioresistance. Some encouraging results have been reported but there have been practical difficulties in producing beams of high enough energy to be adequately penetrating, and of sufficient dose intensity to avoid very long treatment times. There have also been substantial problems arising from increased damage to normal tissues.

### Radiation dose

The commonly used unit of radiation dose absorbed in tissue is the *centiGray* (cGy) which is identical to the previously used rad and is defined as 100 ergs of energy per gramme. The basic SI unit is the *Gray* (Gy): 1 Gy = 100 cGy.

The strength of an isotopic source of radiation is defined in terms of the number of atoms of the isotope which disintegrate per second. The curie was the basic unit prior to the introduction of SI units and was defined as $3.7 \times 10^{10}$ disintegrations per second (1 millicurie (mCi) equals $3.7 \times 10^7$ disintegrations per second). The SI working unit is now the *megabecquerel* (MBq). (1 megabecquerel = $1 \times 10^6$ disintegrations per second = 1/37 curies and 1 gigabecquerel (GBq) = 1000 MBq = 27 mCi.)

# Teletherapy

Much external radiotherapy, particularly palliative treatment, is technically very simple; quite often only a single beam of treatment is required. The position of entry and the size of the beam to be used are marked on the skin by the prescribing doctor, on the basis of clinical or radiological findings and anatomy. The radiographers can then position both the patient and the treatment machine appropriately, prior to switching on for the time required to deliver the prescribed dose. On megavoltage machines, correct positioning is facilitated by the machine producing a beam of light which corresponds to the treatment beam. With orthovoltage machines the field is often defined by applicators of various sizes. The applicator is often shaped rather like an ice-cream cornet with the narrow end attached to the 'head' of the treatment machine and the other end applied to the body surface.

Megavoltage treatment machines are so-called 'isocentric' units. This refers to the ability to rotate the source of irradiation through 360° around a defined point, the isocentre. The patient can be positioned on the treatment couch such that the volume of tissue to be irradiated (treatment volume) has its centre at the machine isocentre. Many isocentric treatments, particularly palliative ones, are also technically simple, incorporating only two beams which enter from exactly opposite sides of the body, in what is known as a 'parallel opposed' arrangement. Such a technique enables the delivery of a higher dose to deep-seated tumours with less damage to more superficial tissues, and with greater dose homogeneity, than would be the case if the tumour was treated to the same dose with a single beam.

## Radiation dose distribution in tissues

The dose of irradiation delivered to tissues falls off as a beam penetrates deeper from the surface. This is because of both increasing distance from the source of the radiation (inverse square law) and absorption of energy from the beam in the more superficial tissues (attenuation). The penetration of X-rays and γ-rays is greater with increasing energy and treatment beams from megavoltage units can deliver a far higher dose to deep-seated tumours than orthovoltage X-rays (for the same dose at or near the surface).

Because of the mechanism of energy transfer to the tissues, superficial and orthovoltage X-rays give a maximum (100 per cent) dose on the skin surface, whilst megavoltage rays exhibit a 'skin sparing' phenomenon. A beam from a 4 meV linear accelerator delivers substantially less than the maximal dose on the surface and the 100 per cent dose is reached only at about a depth of one centimetre. The 100 per cent dose is deeper still with higher energy beams (e.g. 2 cm at 8 meV). This skin-sparing effect results in much less radiation skin

damage than was previously encountered when deep-seated
tumours were treated with orthovoltage beams.

## Physics planning

In some more complicated (usually radical) treatments three
or four beams are used, or two beams which are not parallel-
opposed. These beams intersect to give a high dose to the
treatment volume whilst a substantially lower dose is given to
the surrounding normal tissues outside the volume of in-
tersection, thereby helping to maximise the therapeutic ratio.
Sometimes, in order to produce a homogeneous distribution of
radiation dose throughout the treatment volume, it is necessary preferentially to reduce the intensity of one side of the
treatment beam(s) by the insertion of a lead 'wedge'. This
wedge is placed in the beam in the treatment machine head.

The plans for such treatments, which give radiographers
details of the radiation field sizes, angles of entry, couch
position, dose, wedge usage and other factors, are
normally drawn up by physicists or radiographers using
treatment-planning computers. As well as giving these
instructions the plan contains a graphic representation of a
cross-section through the body at the level of the treatment
volume, on which is indicated the position and size of the
treatment volume as chosen by the oncologist. Superimposed
on this are several lines called isodose lines (the radiotherapeutic equivalent of isobars and isotherms) which join up
points receiving equal radiation doses with the given beam
sizes and angles. The plan is examined before the start of
treatment to check that the dose distribution to the tumour
and its surrounding normal tissues is satisfactory.

## The simulator

This is essential for the degree of accuracy that many treatments require. It is a diagnostic X-ray machine which incorporates a couch on which the patient lies. The relationship
of the X-ray source to the couch can be adjusted to be exactly
the same as on any megavoltage treatment machine. In an
adjacent room there is a television screen on which is displayed the radiographic image of the exposed part of the patient.

Sometimes the tumour is visible on the screen, as in the case of lung cancer or when simulating a bony structure. Sometimes it is necessary to use contrast materials to aid visualisation, as in patients with bladder tumours. Also displayed are cursor lines of a square or rectangle that can be adjusted to correspond to the required treatment volume or beam.

The size and position of the required treatment volume (2 planes) or single beam (1 plane) are adjusted in accordance with the judgement of the doctor planning the treatment. Like the treatment machine there is a light beam corresponding to the X-ray beam, and the margins of any selected beam or treatment volume are also projected on to the patient. These can then be marked either on the patient's skin or on the surface of a transparent plastic mould (see below); the treatment beam can then be set up to the same marks.

The simulator is also often used for *verification*. Once all stages of treatment planning are complete, the accuracy of the treatment plan that is about to start may be checked on the simulator. Accuracy may also be verified during the course of treatment.

## Immobilisation moulds or shells ('jigs')

These also contribute to treatment accuracy and are particularly used in radiotherapy to the head and neck, where high doses need to be given to volumes which are often very close to relatively radiosensitive normal tissues such as the eye and spinal cord. A transparent plastic mould of the surface anatomy is manufactured, usually using a machine which vacuum sucks and heat softens a sheet of plastic over a previously made plaster of Paris impression. During simulation and treatment the mould fits closely over the patient, and is fixed to the couch. This device thus prevents patient movement and allows the size and position of treatment beams to be marked without resorting to skin marks.

## Skin marks

The marks made on patients when moulds are not being used may need to last several weeks during a course of radiotherapy. Marks initially made with a felt-tip pen are often reinforced with silver nitrate, thus producing more sustained marking. Sometimes very small pin-point tattoos are used to define certain points crucial to the accurate setting up of the patient for treatment. A tattoo may also be used as a permanent reference point to delineate a given treatment volume which is especially important if there is a possibility of further radiotherapy to a contiguous area. Where only felt-tip pen marking has been used it is essential that the patient should be told not to wash the marks off.

## Treatment prescription (time, dose and fractionation)

Palliative radiotherapy is usually given in relatively low dosage and over a relatively short time, e.g. 20 Gy (2000 cGy) in 5 consecutive daily treatments (fractions) or 30 Gy in 10 fractions. Palliative radiotherapy for bone pain is often given in a single fraction of 8–10 Gy. Single high dose treatments, given with radical intent, were found (except in some skin treatments) to cause totally unacceptable normal tissue damage and most radical treatments are now fractionated over 3–6 weeks, treating daily, Monday to Friday.

Although there is some evidence that larger fraction sizes (doses) given in shorter overall treatment times have a tendency to cause more long-term normal tissue damage, in practice there is little hard evidence indicating a difference in therapeutic ratio between 3-week and 6-week regimens. However the total dose has to be somewhat reduced when the overall treatment time is shortened, for example 50 Gy in 15 daily fractions over 3 weeks is roughly equivalent to 60 Gy in 30 daily fractions over 6 weeks. The various schedules used (and there is still very wide national and international variation) can be compared, albeit with some limitations, using time, dose and fractionation (TDF) tables. Attempts are being made to compare schedules more accurately by using mathematical models of radiation effects, but these have yet to be established in clinical practice.

Radical radiotherapy is given in high dosage but at a level where the incidence of serious side effects is usually less than 5 per cent, e.g. 50 Gy in 15 fractions, 55 Gy in 20 fractions or 60 Gy in 30 fractions for overt carcinomas. Slightly lower doses are used when treatment is being given adjuvantly for microscopic disease, and lower doses are also given for very radiosensitive non-carcinomatous tumours, e.g. 35–40 Gy in 20 fractions for Hodgkin's disease. Accumulated clinical experience over many decades has led to treatment regimens which are thought to represent the optimal balance between tumour and normal tissue damage.

## Altered fractionation

Radiotherapy has traditionally been given daily, five times per week. Although the reason for this has been principally social it has often been held to be justified by the belief that normal cell repopulation can take place by mitosis on Saturday and Sunday. Dose and fractionation regimens have been developed empirically using five-fraction-per-week schedules. Although normal cell repopulation undoubtedly takes place at weekends (and in between the daily treatment fractions), there is radiobiological evidence to suggest that malignant cells can repopulate to a greater extent. This has led to altered fractionation regimens involving *acceleration* (shorter overall treatment time), *hyperfractionation* (treating more than once per day) or both: the acronym CHART has been used to describe a radical regimen of Continuous (no weekend gap) Hyperfractionated Accelerated Radio-Therapy involving irradiation three times per day over 12 days. There has to be a 5–6- hour gap between fractions to allow normal tissue DNA repair. Individual fraction size is also reduced, and this is expected to result in less normal tissue damage. There is early evidence to suggest that this approach may lead to increased tumour control, with equivalent or reduced late normal tissue damage.

## Radiosensitisers

In an attempt to circumvent radioresistance due to tumour cell hypoxia, trials of radiotherapy given in hyperbaric oxygen were performed. The results were somewhat conflicting, but in the case of head and neck cancer there was good evidence of an improved therapeutic ratio. However the magnitude of the improvement was not thought to justify the expense, logistical difficulties and other problems (e.g. the necessity for ear drum grommets; claustrophobia; risk of explosion) from adopting such treatment as routine. Instead, a variety of compounds have been tried as radiosensitising drugs; their electron-affinity being theoretically capable of increasing the radiosensitivity of hypoxic cells. So far, however, there has been difficulty in administering adequate doses without serious side effects. There have been hints of activity but no proof of benefit. Less toxic compounds with greater electron affinity are now under evaluation.

# Brachytherapy

Brachytherapy can involve the placing of solid (and sealed) radioactive isotopes within body cavities (e.g. the uterus and vagina). This procedure is known as an intracavitary *insertion* and caesium ($^{137}$Cs) is usually used. Placement within solid neoplastic tissue (e.g. needles or wires pushed into tongue or breast carcinomas) is termed an interstitial *implant*, and iridium ($^{192}$Ir) is the most commonly used isotope for this. Isotopes may also be placed very near to the skin within a specially designed and fixed container known as a skin or surface *mould*. Brachytherapy, where feasible, appropriate and well performed, can confer an improved therapeutic ratio over external radiotherapy by delivering a high dose of radiation immediately around the source(s) (in the tumour), with a rapid fall-off in dose a short distance further away in the surrounding normal tissues.

## Remote afterloading

In the past, insertions, implants and surface mould treatments inevitably involved the medical and nursing staff being irradiated. Although the dose received was always monitored and kept within established safety limits, it is now universally thought desirable to keep staff radiation exposure as low as possible and thus in recent years there has been a marked increase in the use of remote afterloading techniques. Here the operator inserts or implants not the radioactive sources themselves, but hollow tube containers of varying diameter:

much smaller diameter tubes are used for implants (inserted with needle trochars inside them which are then removed) than for gynaecological insertions. When the position of the containers is satisfactory (X-rays are often taken to check this, and for dose calculations to be made by the physicist) the tubes are connected to a lead-lined safe which contains the radioactive sources. These are then propelled into position using compressed air, and sucked back at the end of treatment or when the treatment is interrupted, for example for nursing care or meals. Treatment is given in a special, relatively radiation-proof room and proceeds only when there is no-one but the patient(s) in the room. Negligible amounts of radiation escape through the lead lining of the safe and thus the ward staff as well as the theatre staff are almost completely protected.

As with traditional brachytherapy, from the position, number and radiation strengths of the sources the departmental physicist is able to calculate the dose of irradiation given to a specific point or isodose line per unit time. The oncologist prescribes the total dose to be given and the after-loading machine is then programmed to finish treatment automatically once the required treatment time has been completed.

## Other internal uses of isotopes

The very limited penetration of the low energy β-particles emitted by some isotopes makes them suitable for systemic or intracavitary administration. This property is used to enhance the therapeutic ratio by increasing the delivery of irradiation preferentially to certain tissues.

Orally administered radioactive iodine is preferentially taken up in thyroid tissue and sometimes in thyroid carcinoma. The β-particles can deliver a high dose of irradiation to the thyroid tissue with a negligible contribution to other tissues. The γ-rays also released by $^{131}$I penetrate far more deeply and are responsible for some whole body irradiation and radiation leaving the body (which is useful for showing the site(s) and strength of isotope uptake on a gamma-camera picture); this effect is relatively small by comparison with that of the β-particles. Similarly, intravenously administered radioactive phosphorus is preferentially taken up by rapidly dividing bone marrow cells and is thus useful in the treatment of some haematological neoplasms, particularly polycy-thaemia rubra vera. The relatively large particles of colloidal radioactive gold are retained in body cavities into which they are injected, e.g. the peritoneal or pleural cavities. The β-particle component ensures that the main effect of the irradiation is just on the surface of the peritoneum or pleura.

# Radiation protection

For hospital staff and members of the public, concern about radiation exposure centres on carcinogenesis and teratogenesis. Although the risks from low levels of hospital exposure are exceedingly small, particularly when compared with exposure to natural background (particularly cosmic) radiation, there is no known dose threshold for risk and thus all exposure should be kept As Low As is Reasonably Achievable (the 'ALARA' principle). In the United Kingdom guidance is given in the *Guidance Notes For The Protection Of Persons Against Ionising Radiations Arising From Medical And Dental Use* available from HMSO, and in each department there is a Radiation Protection Advisor and a Radiation Safety Committee and Officer(s).

Radiation exposure is kept low by the following procedures:

1 *Shielding of individuals from the source*. This is incorporated in the design of machinery and buildings (lead, thick concrete, etc.).
2 *Increasing the distance from the source*. The inverse square law is an extremely important component of radiation protection.
3 *Reducing the duration of exposure*.

## The film badge

Another important aspect of radiation protection is the monitoring of exposure of individuals, usually using 'film badges' worn at chest or waist level. These contain X-ray film and the amount of radiation is determined by the degree of blackening of the film. They are usually changed every 2–4 weeks and the individual and cumulative measurements recorded. The detection of excessive exposure is important to the individual concerned since further exposure can then be limited. Very occasionally it is of medicolegal relevance and is obviously also important in relation to the detection of risk to other staff.

## Maximum Permissible Dose (MPD)

The dose limit set for occupationally exposed workers is very low, but is somewhat higher than that set for the general population. This is partly practical and partly because any theoretical damage to the genetic pool will be very substantially diluted as occupationally exposed people form such a small percentage of the total population. It is important to stress that any genetic damage is theoretical: no increase in congenital abnormality has been identified in the children of patients treated with radiotherapy or of atomic bomb survivors, providing the radiation exposure was prior to conception. The maximum permissible whole body dose for occupationally exposed persons is 50 milliSieverts (mSv), where the Sievert is the dose of any ionisation which is biologically equivalent to 1 Gray of X-rays. For some ionisations the radiation dose is multiplied by a quality factor to take account of the density of the type of radiation, for example with neutron irradiation the Sievert represents the dose in Grays multiplied by ten. 50 mSv is equivalent to 5 cGy from X- or γ-rays.

# Management of radiation reactions

During and immediately after radiotherapy it is only the acute radiation effects that are troublesome: chronic effects usually become apparent only months or even years later. For most patients some radiation reaction is inevitable, although it is often very mild, particularly with low dose palliative treatment. For all acute reactions the most effective healer is

*Radiation reactions and their management*

| Reaction | Site of Radiation | Management | | |
|---|---|---|---|---|
| | | *Prophylaxis* | *Therapy* | |
| Alopecia | anywhere (irradiated area only!) | (some advocate shaving prior to treatment to reduce follicle dose by lessening 'build up') | reassurance if appropriate (usually recovers after mild to moderate dose) | |
| Cystitis | pelvis | good fluid intake | treat infection (quite often superadded) | |
| Dermatitis | anywhere, but especially with radical treatment to skin folds and naturally moist areas | avoid friction<br>keep open to air where possible<br>avoid washing affected area (particularly when reaction apparent)<br>avoid perfumes and anti-perspirants and preparations containing metal (can cause worse reaction due to 'secondary radiation') | bland talcum powder without metallic content or perfume (e.g. Boots baby powder)<br>emollients (e.g. E45)<br>0.5 per cent aqueous gentian violet solution to areas of moist desquamation | |
| Diarrhoea | abdomen/pelvis | low residue diet; avoid fruit | codeine phosphate<br>kaolin<br>loperamide<br>good fluid intake<br>? interrupt treatment (especially if very severe and/or peritonism) | |

| | | | |
|---|---|---|---|
| Lethargy | almost anywhere except localised superficial | | reassurance |
| Leucocytopenia | any very large volume | monitoring | ? interrupt treatment |
| Mucositis | mouth pharynx oesophagus | stop smoking; avoid irritant and hot foods and drinks good fluid intake | regular mildly antiseptic mouthwashes aspirin rinses/gargles anaesthetic lozenges benzydamine oral rinse (Difflam) treat candida (a common complication) antacid/topical anaesthetic mixture (e.g. Mucaine) ? interrupt treatment |
| Nausea/vomiting | any large volume but especially abdomen or pelvis: spinal irradiation may exit through abdomen | occasionally anti-emetics | metoclopramide prochlorperazine domperidone |
| Thrombocyto-penia | any very large volume | monitoring | ? interrupt treatment |

time, as they are virtually always self-limiting. However
there is often much that can be done prophylactically and
therapeutically to make the patient more comfortable as
shown in the Table on pages 56 and 57.

## NOTES

# CHAPTER 7

# Drug Treatment

Although the currently available anti-cancer drugs are often capable of killing a proportion of the total number of malignant cells in a patient, by themselves they are capable only of eradicating a small percentage of cancers. Curative potential seems to be largely confined to relatively uncommon tumours. However, there is evidence that anti-cancer drugs may be capable of eradicating relatively small numbers of metastatic and locally residual cells in certain patients with some of the more common tumours, when given in addition to local treatment with surgery or radiotherapy. Given in this way ('adjuvantly') the evidence of benefit is strongest for breast carcinoma and some paediatric malignancies.

In routine clinical practice anti-cancer drugs fall into two main groups, hormonal and cytotoxic. Hormonal agents are generally much better tolerated than cytotoxic drugs which can cause severe morbidity and even death. Attention to dosage, absorption, metabolism and excretion is particularly important with cytotoxics. For all drug treatment efficacy depends not only on the innate sensitivity of a particular tumour, but also on the extent to which that sensitivity exists in all of the tumour cells and the ability of the malignant cells to acquire resistance. The delivery of adequate amounts of the drug to those cells via blood vessels, and very occasionally by other routes (intrathecal; intraperitoneal; intrapleural), is also crucial.

## Starting drug treatment

Before starting any drug treatment the following are mandatory:

1 Clarification of the aim of treatment.

59

2 Discussion of rationale and any common side effects with patient.

3 Documentation of pre-treatment tumour burden. This includes measurement of palpable or visible tumours, and X-rays and photographs where relevant and helpful.

4 Check that recent full blood count, blood urea (creatinine clearance for some nephrotoxic drugs, e.g. cisplatinum) and liver function are normal prior to cytotoxic chemotherapy. Abnormalities may prohibit treatment or dictate dose modification.

5 Check that proposed dose and route of administration is correct, and in particular check that the quantity of cytotoxic drug specified in the treatment regimen refers to the absolute dose or the dose per surface area or weight.

6 Check that general health does not contraindicate treatment, e.g. history of thromboembolism in patient being offered stilboestrol or of heart failure in patient being considered for adriamycin.

7 Check that other medication is not likely to interact (see list).

8 Advise patient about possible serious side effects and appropriate action if potentially sinister symptoms occur, particularly the risk of serious infection and haemorrhage (including petechiae) in patients on cytotoxic chemotherapy.

9 Read the manufacturer's data sheet(s) unless already familiar with the drug(s) proposed.

The following are also rather important:

1 Try to give the patient a good idea of the probable or possible duration of treatment.

2 Make arrangements for the provision of a wig where alopecia is likely and the patient would like one.

## Continuing drug treatment

There can be no justification for continuing any treatment for cancer in the face of persistent tumour growth, and there may be little justification for continuing in the face of significant toxicity if the treatment intent is palliative. Close monitoring of efficacy is particularly important with cytotoxic chemotherapy, because of its toxicity. Before continuing with drug treatment the following are mandatory:

1 Assessment of response. It is very rarely justified to continue with treatment if there is evidence of continued tumour growth. If the disease is static or only slightly responding continuation of treatment may be justified, but usually not if there is severe toxicity.

2 Assessment of toxicity, subjective and objective. Check if there are any mandatory investigations for monitoring of toxicity. Enquire about any other new symptoms which may be side effects but which the patient may not attribute to treatment, e.g. vincristine peripheral neuropathy. Toxicity may justify stopping, delaying, or modifying treatment. The full blood count must be checked immediately prior to every pulse of cytotoxic chemotherapy and trends in cell concentrations must be looked at as well as absolute levels.

# Hormonal Drugs

The relative lack of toxicity of hormonal drugs makes then attractive treatment options for those patients who have malignancies which are known sometimes to be susceptible to endocrine manoeuvres. Such maneouvres include surgical or radiotherapeutic endocrine ablation as well as drugs.

These drugs comprise hormones and anti-hormones. Their mode of action is imperfectly understood although their efficacy probably depends on the presence of hormone receptors on the malignant cell surface. Beneficial withdrawal responses are sometimes seen when administration of a hormonal agent is stopped on relapse following a prior response of usually long duration. Hormonal drugs do not have curative potential by themselves, but it is possible that they may sometimes have curative potential when given adjuvantly with effective local treatment.

*Summary of principal endocrine agents used in the treatment of cancer*

| Drug | Definition/action | Main side effects | Dose | Activity |
|---|---|---|---|---|
| Aminoglutethimide (Orimeten) | blocks endogenous oestrogen production (adrenal & peripheral tissue) | drowsiness & rash (usually subside if continued) hypoadrenalism rarely agranulocytosis | 250 mg bd orally – steroid supplement essential e.g. hydrocortisone 20 mg bd | breast prostate |
| Cyproterone (Cyprostat) | anti-androgen | fatigue thromboembolism gynaecomastia rarely liver damage | 6 × 50 mg tablets per day | prostate |
| Estramustine (Estracyt) | oestrogen bound to mustine (cytotoxic) | nausea gynaecomastia thromboembolism | 4 × 140 mg capsules per day | prostate |
| Fosfestrol (Honvan) | oestrogen which is inert until activated by tissue phosphatase | perineal pain nausea/vomiting fluid retention | 10–20 ml IV daily for one week 3 × 100 mg tables per day | prostate |
| Goserelin (Zoladex) | LHRH analogue | hot flushes gynaecomastia | 3.6 mg subcutaneously in anterior abdominal | prostate breast |

| | | initial tumour stimulation – beware spinal cord compression | wall<br>initial anti-androgen therapy advisable for prostate carcinoma | |
|---|---|---|---|---|
| Medroxy-progesterone | progestogen | increased appetite and sense of well-being weight gain | 400–1000 mg per day (depending on bioavailability) | breast endometrium (kidney) |
| Megestrol | progestogen | as above | 160 mg per day | as above |
| Nandrolone (Durabolin) | anabolic | virilisation fluid retention hypercalcaemia | 25–50 mg IM per week | breast |
| Stilboestrol | oestrogen | nausea/vomiting fluid retention thromboembolism | 15 mg per day in 1–3 mg per day in | breast prostate |
| Tamoxifen | anti-oestrogen | nausea fluid retention hypercalcaemia warfarin toxicity | 20–40 mg per day (no benefit from >20 mg post-menopausally) | breast (endometrium) (ovary) |
| Thyroxine | | | adequate to suppress TSH secretion, usually .2-.3 mg/day (40–60 µg T3) | thyroid |

Tumours which may show a response to endocrine manoeuvres

> Prostate carcinoma
> Breast carcinoma (female and male)
> Endometrial carcinoma
> Thyroid carcinoma (differentiated)
> Ovarian carcinoma (rarely)
> Renal carcinoma (rarely)

# Cytotoxic Drugs

These drugs are usually considerably more toxic than hormonal drugs. They preferentially affect dividing cells in tumours and their hosts, and the side effects are often most apparent in those tissues or organs where there is a rapid cell turnover. These include the bone marrow, gastrointestinal epithelium and hair follicles.

A cytotoxic drug usually exerts its effect by one or more of the following:

1 Interfering with the production of DNA (e.g. antimetabolites such as methotrexate and 5-fluorouracil).
2 Damaging already formed DNA (e.g. alkylating agents such as cyclophosphamide and melphalan, antibiotics such as adriamycin and actinomycin D, nitrosoureas such as BCNU and CCNU).
3 Damaging the mitotic spindle (e.g. vinca alkaloids such as vincristine and vinblastine).

Some drugs are described as being 'cycle specific' and are effective throughout the cell cycle (e.g. the alkylating agents and adriamycin) while others are called 'phase specific' and exert their effect at a particular phase of the cycle (e.g. methotrexate is effective during DNA synthesis and vincristine during mitosis).

Cytotoxic drugs may be given singly or in combination. The rationale for combinations is a reduction in either innate or acquired drug resistance. The majority of all cancers are innately resistant to the drugs presently available and most malignant tumours that are initially sensitive will eventually acquire resistance if they are not eradicated. Many tumours will show an initial response to chemotherapy but eventually regrow as a result of the continued multiplication of an initially small population of innately resistant cells. With the exception of one tumour, choriocarcinoma – the only malignant tumour which is known to be antigenically foreign (due to the paternal genetic contribution) the use of combinations rather than single drugs is essential for cure. Effective combination chemotherapy usually incorporates individual drugs which act in different ways, and which have different toxicity profiles. The aim is to improve the therapeutic ratio by using drugs at slightly lower doses than if they were being used singly, and thus reduce the probability that any particular toxicity will become prohibitive.

Chemotherapy can be beneficial only if it is disproportionately toxic to malignant cells compared with normal cells. Pulses of chemotherapy are empirically timed to ensure sufficient recovery of the normal cell population so that the next course can be given with reasonable safety. The interval between courses differs for different regimens but the most common interval is 3 weeks. The degree of recovery of normal tissue damage is principally assessed by measuring the full blood count, which reflects the extent of recovery of the bone marrow – one of the most sensitive of normal tissues. Cytotoxic chemotherapy should never be given without an up-to-date measurement of the full blood count and when there is leucopenia the differential count is also important. For both curative and palliative treatment, host factors very substantially influence the final outcome. Frailty, advancing age, altered metabolism and impaired excretion may greatly impair tolerance to chemotherapy.

## Potentially curative chemotherapy

This tends to be justifiably more toxic than treatment given with palliative intent: some regimens are exceedingly toxic. The number of cells (malignant and normal) killed by a dose of a cytotoxic drug is related to the dose given. For most cytotoxic treatments there is good clinical evidence of a dose response, and more aggressive regimens tend to be associated with a higher chance of tumour eradication. However, some of the most aggressive combinations stand a considerable chance of causing death and the balance drawn between the attempt to cure and the attempt to avoid serious toxicity depends not only on the characteristics of the individual patient but also on the philosophy of the individual oncologist.

Several cycles of chemotherapy are required for cure. Each cycle or 'pulse' tends to kill an approximately equal fraction of the malignant cell population, thus a pulse which reduced the cell population from 1,000,000 to 10,000 might be expected, when repeated, to reduce the cell population from 10,000 to 100. Since only 1 cm$^3$ of tumour contains approximately $10^9$ cells, it is usually necessary to continue giving curative chemotherapy for some time after all clinical evidence of active disease has disappeared.

## Palliative chemotherapy

Since this is given with the aim of the relief of symptoms, or the prolongation of enjoyable life, severe toxicity defeats the object. For many common cancers the response rates are low and often it is not easy to justify attempts to achieve responses for a minority at the expense of toxicity and no benefit for the majority. Mere diminution of tumour bulk, although essential for the contemporary definition of 'response', is often the least important end-point for the patient. Even where some symptomatic relief is achieved patients may sometimes feel that it did not justify the side effects and time away from home. There is considerably more variation in oncologists' philosophy concerning palliation than there is for potentially curative treatment.

## Malignancies for which cytotoxic chemotherapy can be curative or contribute to cure

> Choriocarcinoma
> Ewing's sarcoma
> Germ cell tumours of testis and ovary (teratoma, seminoma, dysgerminoma)
> Hodgkin's disease
> Acute leukaemia

Non-Hodgkin's lymphoma
Embryonal rhabdomyosarcoma
Wilm's tumour

**Malignancies for which cytotoxic chemotherapy is of considerable efficacy and may possibly have curative potential**

Breast carcinoma (possible curative potential for adjuvant treatment only)
Neuroblastoma
Osteogenic sarcoma (possible curative potential for adjuvant treatment only)
Ovarian carcinoma (possible curative potential for adjuvant treatment only)
Small cell (oat cell) lung carcinoma

**Malignancies for which cytotoxic chemotherapy has considerable palliative potential**

Breast carcinoma
Cervical carcinoma
Head and neck squamous carcinoma
Chronic leukaemia
Myeloma
Ovarian carcinoma
Small cell (oat cell) lung carcinoma

## Intravenous administration

### Drug preparation

Whenever possible cytotoxic drugs should be reconstituted and drawn up in a laminar air flow cabinet by specially trained staff. A laminar air flow cabinet prevents the inhalation by staff of drug aerosols, which are easily created when drugs are drawn up. Several studies have shown that the urine of staff reconstituting and drawing up cytotoxic drugs outside laminar air flow cabinets is mutagenic *in vitro*, and there is legitimate concern about possible carcinogenicity and teratogenicity. The reconstitution and drawing up of cytotoxic drugs is now increasingly done in dedicated units within hospital pharmacies. However, it is still often necessary for drugs to be prepared for injection outside dedicated units and without laminar air flow cabinets. Ideally a specially designated relatively remote area should be used, and this should not be close to air conditioning or heating ducts. No one should reconstitute and draw up cytotoxic drugs without appropriate training and without having consulted the manufacturer's data sheet. The compatibility of the drug with the proposed diluent and with any other intravenous fluid must also be checked.

Cytotoxic drugs should be prepared on a smooth work surface, ideally paper covered. Gloves, mask, goggles and a coat with long sleeves should be worn and the whole procedure carried out in an unhurried manner, with great care. This minimises the risk of possible potentially hazardous spills, contamination of skin or eyes and aerosol formation. 'Closed' systems should be used for reconstitution whenever possible and glass ampoules should be covered with a swab before breaking open. Positive or negative pressures within rubber-capped containers should be avoided either by venting (putting another needle just through the rubber top) or by correct syringe technique. The use of large-bore needles helps to lessen pressure differentials and Luer locks should be used on all syringes. All the waste must be put in a 'sharps' container for incineration.

## Injection

No one should administer cytotoxic drugs without proper training. The patient's other medication should always be known before administration, and the possibility of interaction borne in mind. Anaphylaxis is very rare, but can occur with a variety of drugs.

Several intravenous cytotoxic drugs can cause very severe tissue damage if even very small amounts are extravasated during or after the injection. Such damage occasionally requires plastic surgery, sometimes of an extensive nature. The adequacy of access should be confirmed prior to injection, which should always be given via a 'butterfly' or plastic cannula, preferably taped in place, and never through a needle attached directly to the syringe. Whenever possible the antecubital fossa should be avoided, and any other site where early extravasation may not easily be seen. Normal saline should be injected before and after the cytotoxic drug(s) with any anti-emetic injections being given first. The arm cuff must be deflated or removed prior to injection as continued raised venous pressure will predispose to extravasation: a tightly rolled-up shirt or jersey sleeve can have the same effect. Injections must proceed slowly and the injection site should be observed closely throughout the procedure. The patient should be instructed to report any pain at the injection site immediately, and the injection must be interrupted immediately if this occurs, although pain does not necessarily indicate extravasation. Injections in lymphoedematous arms should be avoided.

If extravasation does occur of a vesicant or irritant drug (generally any drug for which there is no available oral preparation) first leave the needle in place, attempt to suck back any drug and then partially inject the recommended antidotes for the drug via the original needle, if still in place. The remainder of the antidote should be injected at several points immediately around the injection site using a very fine needle.

| CYTOTOXIC | ANTIDOTE |
|---|---|
| Adriamycin; epirubicin; daunorubicin; doxorubicin; BCNU | 1 ml hydrocortisone (100 mg/ml) or dexamethasone (4 mg/ml) and 5 ml sodium bicarbonate (8.4 per cent). Also apply ice pack and topical steroid cream. For the anthracyclines also topical 99 per cent DMSO to the affected area 6-hourly for 14 days. |
| Mustine; mithramycin; actinomycin D; mitomycin C | 5 ml sodium thiosulphate (10 per cent). Repeat 3 hourly ×3. Apply ice pack. |
| Vincristine; vinblastine; vindesine; etoposide (VP 16) | 5 ml hyaluronidase (150 units/ml). Repeat 3 hourly ×3. Keep injection site warm. Avoid steroids. |

Superficial thrombophlebitis is quite common after in-travenous injection of cytotoxic drugs. It may be alleviated by heparinoid cream (300 mg/100 g) applied liberally over the affected area three times per day and covered with a dressing. It can be of value when used prophylactically in some patients particularly predisposed to this problem.

## Scalp cooling

Although several cytotoxic drugs do not carry a significant risk of hair loss, this is one of the most widely known and feared side effects of cytotoxic chemotherapy. The possibility of drug-induced partial or total alopecia is very disturbing to some patients, particularly women, despite being reassured that the effect is only temporary and despite the availability of excellent wigs. In routine clinical oncology practice this is often a problem with drug regimens incorporating adriamy-cin or epirubicin in conventional dosage.

Scalp cooling at the time of intravenous administration reduces the metabolism of the hair follicles, and scalp blood supply, thereby reducing toxicity to the hair follicles and the incidence and severity of alopecia. It is particularly feasible for patients receiving adriamycin or epirubicin because of the short plasma half-life of these drugs. A variety of cold-caps are available, usually being in essence double-layered bath-ing-caps filled with cryogel. They are stored in a refrigerator at −15 to −20°C and are applied over wet hair for approx-imately 20 minutes prior to injection and for about 45 minutes afterwards.

Although scalp cooling does substantially reduce alopecia it has been found to be less effective when higher anthracycline dosages are used, and also when liver function is abnormal since this prolongs the plasma half-life. It can also be uncom-fortable and may substantially prolong the time a patient has to spend in the clinic, possibly adding to psychological morbid-ity. It must also not be forgotten that any therapeutic effect of the drug on neoplastic cells in the scalp will also be reduced. Metastatic involvement of the scalp is not uncommon, parti-cularly in patients with breast carcinoma, and this technique is contraindicated in patients receiving potentially curative treatment for leukaemia or non-Hodgkin's lymphoma.

## Right atrial catheters

For some patients requiring prolonged chemotherapy venous access by means of an indwelling silastic right atrial (commonly Hickman) catheter may be extremely helpful, particularly where chemotherapy causes more intense thrombophlebitis and subsequent occlusion, leading to a progressive loss in accessible peripheral venous sites. For some patients (especially children) this is also helpful in circumventing needle phobia. In addition it enables low dose-rate continuous infusion chemotherapy, for which there is some evidence of an improved therapeutic ratio in the treatment of some advanced carcinomas. The Hickman catheter can be used not only for administration of fluids and drugs, but also for the withdrawal of blood samples. There are dual lumen versions which allow flexibility in the administration of drugs and fluids and the simultaneous withdrawal of blood samples, and these are essential if parenteral nutrition is to be given.

The catheter is usually inserted under local anaesthesia but in the sterile surroundings of the theatre. They are usually introduced into the right subclavian or jugular (external or internal) vein via an infraclavicular or low-neck incision respectively. An incision is also made lower down the anterior chest wall enabling the catheter to be tunnelled some way under the skin and subcutaneous tissues, thereby reducing the chance of bacterial infection. There is also a Dacron cuff around the catheter in the subcutaneous tunnel which produces a local fibroblastic reaction and so helps to anchor the catheter, thus providing a barrier against ascending infection. These catheters can be retained fully functionally for long periods of time under careful supervision, even for periods of longer than two years. Patients can resume most normal activity with the catheter in place.

Immediate complications include pneumothorax and haemothorax. Thrombocytopenic patients must receive platelet cover for the procedure, and disseminated intravascular coagulation is an absolute contraindication. Other complications include blockage by clots and central venous thrombosis, and infections involving the subcutaneous tunnel or entry site. Except when being used for continuous low-dose-rate infusion the catheters should be flushed regularly (often once daily but sometimes less frequently) by the nurse, patient or spouse (or other carer at home) with heparinised saline (e.g. 2 ml of 100 units/ml solution). They must be filled with heparin solution after every administration of drugs or blood products, and after every blood sample removal. Meticulous attention must be given to aseptic technique, particularly in patients likely to be, or to become, substantially immunosuppressed. The dressing covering the exit site should be changed at least twice weekly, and an antiseptic ointment (e.g. providone-iodine) applied around the site. Occlusive bacteriocidal dressings are probably not necessary for most patients receiving continuous palliative chemotherapy for carcinoma.

A swab for microbiology must be taken from the entry site if local infection is suspected. In the event of fever, blood cultures should be taken from both a peripheral vein and the catheter. Infections involving the tunnel often require removal of the catheter because of a poor response to antibiotics whereas infection within the catheter itself can usually be treated successfully without removal, antibiotics being administered through it. Blocked catheters can usually be cleared by flushing with heparinised saline ± streptokinase or urokinase, although the dislodged clots must inevitably embolise to the lungs.

The catheter can easily be removed in the clinic or on the ward, by gentle traction following mobilisation of the Dacron cuff through an overlying incision made under local anaesthesia. Pressure should be applied over the track to control bleeding, and the catheter tip should always be sent for culture.

# Toxicity

## Common or significant side effects that can occur with most cytotoxic drugs

Bone marrow suppression
Nausea and vomiting (including anticipatory)

Alopecia [temporary] (especially adriamycin and analogues, cyclophosphamide, mustine, bleomycin, vinca alkaloids and etoposide)
Changes in hair texture and colour (usually temporary)
Malaise
Lethargy
Psychological intolerance (including anxiety and depression)
Altered taste
Impaired appetite
Specific food aversions
Stomatitis
Thrombophlebitis and venous occlusion at injection site
Muscle aching
Amenorrhoea
Infertility
Immunosuppression
Rarely avascular bone necrosis (particularly with steroid-containing regimens)

## Other common or significant side effects of cytotoxic drugs

| Drug | Side Effects, Remedies and Precautions |
| --- | --- |
| Actinomycin D | Potentiates skin and mucous membrane reactions to concurrent or previous (recall reaction) radiotherapy. |
| Adriamycin | Cardiomyopathy (particularly at total dosage >550 mg/m$^2$, with high individual doses and if heart previously irradiated). Radionuclide ejection fraction studies are much more sensitive than electrocardiography and have a rôle in prediction and prevention but are rarely indicated in routine clinical practice.<br>Red urine (warn patient).<br>Dose should be reduced if liver function is impaired (raised bilirubin) |

Bleomycin

Cutaneous, including erythema, hyperpigmentation and hyperkeratosis. Lung – pneumonitis leading to pulmonary fibrosis (especially if previous or concurrent lung irradiation). Fever.

If given IM pain can be prevented by using 1 per cent lignocaine as solvent. Steroids are effective in preventing fever and in improving symptoms in pneumonitis (but probably not effective in preventing fibrosis).

High oxygen concentrations under anaesthesia can cause lung toxicity in patients treated pre-operatively with bleomycin.

Reduce dose if renal function impaired.
Total dose of 500 mg should not normally be exceeded.

Busulphan

Pulmonary fibrosis: steroids may improve symptoms. Myelosuppression may be delayed. Hepatic nodular regeneration and portal hypertension in patients receiving busulphan and thioguanine for chronic myeloid leukaemia.

Carboplatin

Much less symptomatically toxic than its analogue cisplatin. Nausea and vomiting is less severe, nephrotoxicity is much less common and usually only mild: high-volume hydration is not required. Ototoxicity is very much less. However myelosuppression is substantially more severe, particularly in the presence of abnormal renal function.

Carmustine
(BCNU)

Facial flushing. Pain at injection site. Both may be prevented by slow infusion over 1–2 hours. Hepatotoxicity. Lung toxicity with total dose >1,400 mg/m$^2$. Myelosuppression may be delayed.

Cisplatin

Nephrotoxicity. Renal function must be monitored and creatinine clearance must be performed before start of course – serum creatinine levels are often adequate for subsequent pulses. Prophylaxis for nephrotoxicity is forced diuresis with normal saline infusion at a rate of 250 ml/ hour starting 8 hours before and continuing throughout the 6-hour administration of the drug (dissolved in it) and for a total of 24 hours. Urine output must be closely monitored. If output is not at least 200 ml/hour by the start of the administration of the drug, mannitol 12.5 gms should be given IV ± frusemide 40 mg and this may need to be repeated, particularly if there is evidence of fluid overload. It has been suggested that both intravenous sodium thiosulphate and the combination of verapamil and cimetidine may additionally help to protect against cisplatin nephrotoxicity.

Hypomagnesaemia. This is very common but only rarely is it symptomatic. Tetany, paraesthesiae, weakness and dizziness may occur. Magnesium chloride or sulphate should then be added to the infusion – 50 mmol over 12 hours. In some regimens it is given prophylactically in the pre-treatment hydration and also orally in between pulses (see section on hypomagne-saemia).

Ototoxicity, resulting in high frequency loss and/or tinnitus. Impaired hearing of normal conversation is very rare but audiometric monitoring is sometimes appropriate, particularly where evidence of early ototoxicity would justify a switch to carboplatin. Vertigo.

Nausea and vomiting is usually severe. Peripheral neuropathy and Lhermitte's sign are rare side effects.

*Interaction.* Enhanced renal toxicity with aminoglycosides.

**Cyclophosphamide**

Haemorrhagic cystitis. This can be prevented with mesna (see ifosfamide) but this is rarely required. However a good fluid intake and frequent micturition are important. A urine output of 3 litres per day should be achieved for at least 48 hours starting just prior to bolus injections and at least 2 litres per day throughout oral administration.

Hyponatremia (inappropriate ADH secretion) with very high doses.

*Interactions.* Enhanced toxicity with allopurinol. Potentiation of hypoglycaemic drugs.

**Cytosine arabinoside**

Flu-like syndrome – steroids are beneficial. Conjunctivitis – hydrocortisone eye-drops for 10 days may be prophylactic.

| | |
|---|---|
| Dacarbazine (DTIC) | Nausea and vomiting is often severe. The reconstituted solution is sensitive to light and must be protected from it and used quickly: the infusion bag and line should be draped. Flulike syndrome is unusual. |
| Daunorubicin | Cardiomyopathy particularly at total dose $>600$ mg/m$^2$ and if heart previously irradiated or diseased. Radionuclide cardiac studies as for adriamycin. Red urine (warn patient). |
| Epirubicin | Cardiomyopathy particularly at total dose $>1000$ mg/m$^2$ and if heart previously irradiated or diseased. Radionuclide cardiac studies as for adriamycin. Red urine (warn patient). |
| Etoposide (VP16) | Hypotension if infused in under 30 minutes. Hypersensitivity reactions are also seen with bronchospasm, flushing and either hypotension or hypertension. |
| 5-Fluorouracil | Stomatitis. This may be lessened in those previously troubled by prophylactic allopurinol mouthwashes – 900 mg dissolved in 150 ml water for 5 minutes, repeated 4–6 times/day for 6 days starting at the beginning of 5-fluorouracil administration. Diarrhoea, cerebellar syndrome, conjunctivitis, cardiotoxicity: treatment should be discontinued if there is cardiac chest pain or tachyarrhythmia. Dosage should be reduced if there is impaired liver function (raised bilirubin). |

Hydroxyurea

Megaloblastic erythropoiesis (not due to folate or vitamin $B_{12}$ deficiency). Reduce dose if marked renal impairment.

*Interactions.* Drowsiness with antidepressants, alcohol and other CNS depressants.

Ifosfamide

Haemorrhagic cystitis. Mesna prophylaxis is essential and total fluid intake should be at least 3 litres in 24 hours during treatment, and in the 24 hours immediately after. When ifosfamide is fractionated over 5 days (1–2-hour infusion per day) the normal total dose of mesna is 60 per cent of the ifosfamide dose, given IV at 0, 4 and 8 hours (20 per cent each time). When ifosfamide is not fractionated but given as a 24-hour infusion, or more quickly, the normal total dose of mesna is 120 per cent of the ifosfamide dose, 60 per cent being given in equal divided doses at 4-hourly intervals and 60 per cent being given 4 hourly during the 12 hours after ifosfamide administration is completed. This can be given orally: the unpleasant-tasting drug can be mixed in a large quantity of fruit juice. Only minor modifications need to be made if the ifosfamide is given over 30 minutes.
When calculating the mesna dose, each fraction should be rounded up to the nearest whole ampoule (400 mg or 1 gm).
Ifosfamide can exert an anti-diuretic effect and diuretics may be necessary to maintain a good urine output.

Ifosfamide/mesna can cause false +ve ketonuria.

Encephalopathy is a rare side effect, manifested by such as lethargy, confusion, hallucinations, cerebellar signs, seizures and even coma. The risk is substantially increased if there is impaired renal and hepatic function as manifested by serum albumin <40 g/l and serum creatinine >100μmol/l, particularly in the presence of pelvic tumour. Lower levels of albumin and higher levels of creatinine independently confer a significant risk of encephalopathy.

| | |
|---|---|
| Interferons | Flu-like syndrome is very common, including fever, fatigue and myalgia. Its severity can be reduced by evening administration and paracetamol. Vomiting, diarrhoea, hypotension, encephalopathy, peripheral neuropathy, hepatotoxicity, alopecia. |
| Lomustine CCNU | Myelosuppression may be delayed with recovery not until 6 or more weeks. |
| Melphalan | Myelosuppression may be delayed. Dose should be reduced, at least initially, if there is moderate to severe renal impairment. |
| 6-Mercaptopurine | Dosage should be reduced, at least initially, in the presence of moderate to severe renal impairment. |
| | *Interaction.* The dose should also be reduced by at least 50 per cent if the patient is on allopurinol and if at all possible these drugs should not be given concurrently: allopurinol blocks 6-MP metabolism. |

Methotrexate

Mucositis, conjunctivitis, diarrhoea, hepatotoxicity. Renal impairment in high dosage. Cerebral atrophy in conjunction with cranial irradiation. Demyelinating leucoencephalopathy with intrathecal administration.

Dose should be reduced in presence of renal impairment.

The drug can accumulate in moderate to large collections of pleural or ascitic fluid, return slowly to the systemic circulation and cause severe toxicity. These should be tapped or the dosage reduced.

Substantially increased toxicity has also been described in patients given red blood cell transfusions during, or immediately after, intermediate dosage $(50-200 \text{ mg/m}^2)$ methotrexate infusion, and attributed to the transfused cells acting as a reservoir for the drug.

Doses over 80 mg/m$^2$ should be followed by estimation of serum methotrexate levels or the antidote folinic acid given routinely at 24 hours after methotrexate, and subsequently 6-hourly (usually parenterally for $\geq$24 hours), as dictated by the dose of methotrexate or serum methotrexate levels. Estimation of levels is essential at methotrexate doses $>$200 mg/m$^2$. At these higher methotrexate dose levels the urine must be kept alkaline to prevent drug crystal precipitation in the renal tubules. Urinary pH must be monitored and alkalinisation achieved with sodium bicarbonate in the infusion (500 ml 1.4% solution 6 hourly) or orally (5 $\times$ 625 mg tablets every 3 hours) ± oral acetazolamide (500 mg qds). The fluid input should be ⩾3 litres/m$^2$/day. Prehydration and alkalinisation should begin ⩾12 hours prior to methotrexate.

Doses of methotrexate greater than 1 gm should not normally be given if there is impaired renal function. Creatinine clearance must be performed before starting and the serum creatinine estimated before each pulse. Folinic acid is normally given 15–30 mg 6 hourly for 24–48 hours, starting about 24 hours after the start of methotrexate. Oral initial administration is reserved for low doses. For doses >1 g the serum level should be estimated at 24 hours (after start of administration). Higher doses of folinic acid (100–1,000 mg/m$^2$) should be given if levels are >$1 \times 10^{-5}$ m at 24 hours, >$5 \times 10^{-7}$ m at 48 hours or >$1 \times 10^{-7}$ m at 72 hours in order to prevent severe and even life-threatening toxicity. Folinic acid should be continued until the serum methotrexate level is <$5 \times 10^{-8}$ m. The need for higher folinic acid doses is also indicated by a ⩾50% rise in the serum creatinine at 24 hours.

*Interactions.* Aspirin, other non-steroidal anti-inflammatory drugs, sulphonamides, tetracycline, hypoglycaemic drugs and phenytoin may displace drug from binding protein and cause enhanced toxicity. Warfarin may be potentiated.

| | |
|---|---|
| Mitomycin C | Myelosuppression may be delayed with nadir at 6 or more weeks after injection. Haemolysis. |
| | Severe renal toxicity is a rare side effect – blood urea should be measured before each pulse above the threshold accumulative dose, and the urine checked for blood and protein. This carries a significant mortality risk. The threshold accumulative dose is quite low $(30 \, \text{mg/m}^2)$. Haemolysis may respond to plasmapharesis or extracorporeal immunoabsorption of immune complexes. |
| Mitozantrone | Cardiomyopathy particularly above $160 \, \text{mg/m}^2$ and if adriamycin, epirubicin, daunorubicin or cardiac radiotherapy have been given previously or if there was previous cardiac disease. |
| | Blue/green urine (warn patient). Onycholysis. |
| Mustine | Must be given within 15 minutes of preparation of the solution as stability is rapidly lost. |
| Procarbazine | Alcohol intolerance resembling disulfiram reaction. Patients must be warned of this. This drug is a monoamine oxidase inhibitor and tyramine-rich foods should also be avoided. |
| Retinoids | Desquamation, erythema, alopecia, dry or ulcerated mucous membranes. Hepatotoxicity, headache, ataxia, hypertriglyceridaemia. |
| Semustine (methyl CCNU) | Renal failure. This is a cumulative toxicity and the total dose should not |

exceed 1,200 mg/m$^2$. Marrow toxicity can be delayed and prolonged.

6-Thioguanine
Stomatitis, diarrhoea, hepatotoxicity. Consider dose reduction if impaired liver or renal function. See busulphan.

Thiotepa
Dose should be reduced with impaired renal function.

Treosulfan
Tablets should be swallowed whole to avoid stomatitis.

Vinblastine
Constipation due to autonomic neuropathy – lactulose is helpful. Jaw pain. Hyponatraemia due to inappropriate ADH secretion. Transient early onset thrombocytopenia is common, and is due to peripheral platelet destruction, not marrow toxicity.

Vincristine
Peripheral and autonomic neuropathy, the latter causing constipation – lactulose is helpful. Hyponatraemia due to inappropriate ADH secretion. Jaw pain.

*Interaction.* Enhanced peripheral neuropathy with isoniazid.

Vindesine
Largely as for vinblastine and vincristine: peripheral neuropathy risk intermediate.

**Notable drug interactions**

Alcohol
Enhanced drowsiness with hydroxyurea
Antabuse effect with procarbazine

Allopurinol
Enhanced cyclophosphamide, azathioprine and 6-mercaptopurine toxicity

| | |
|---|---|
| Aminoglycosides | Enhanced renal toxicity from cisplatin |
| Anti-coagulants | Enhanced or reduced efficacy may be seen in patients receiving cytotoxic chemotherapy. Enhanced toxicity with tamoxifen. Closer monitoring is advisable |
| Anti-depressants (tricyclic) | Enhanced drowsiness with hydroxyurea |
| Anti-emetics | Enhanced drowsiness with hydroxyurea |
| Anti-inflammatory drugs (non-steroidal) | Enhanced methotrexate toxicity |
| Aspirin | Enhanced methotrexate toxicity |
| Chloramphenicol | Reduced cyclophosphamide efficacy |
| Cimetidine | Enhanced marrow damage from carmustine (BCNU) |
| CNS depressants | Potentiation by hydroxyurea |
| Frusemide | Enhanced renal toxicity from cisplatin |
| Hypoglycaemic agents | Potentiation by cyclophosphamide Reduced efficacy with asparaginase |
| Insulin | Potentiation by cyclophosphamide |
| Isoniazid | Enhanced peripheral toxicity from vincristine |
| Oxygen | Higher anaesthetic concentrations may precipitate pulmonary fibrosis from bleomycin |
| Probenecid | Enhanced methotrexate toxicity |
| Suxamethonium | Enhanced activity leading to prolonged apnoea, with cyclophosphamide |

Vaccines            Live vaccines may result in very se-
                    vere infections in patients receiving
                    cytotoxic chemotherapy. These in-
                    clude measles, polio, rubella and yel-
                    low fever.

# Bone Marrow Transplantation

Transplantation of bone marrow (BMT) enables the administration of aggressive treatment with cytotoxic chemotherapy
with or without whole body irradiation, which would otherwise cause profound or fatal toxicity due to marrow suppression. The transfused marrow is either the recipient's own
marrow, removed prior to treatment (autologous BMT), that
taken from an HLA (human leukocyte antigen) identical
donor who is not an identical twin (allogeneic BMT), or that
taken from an identical twin (syngeneic). Marrow ablative
treatment followed by BMT is of established potentially curative value in the management of patients with acute
leukaemias and chronic granulocytic leukaemia. In patients
with acute leukaemia the therapeutic ratio is highest if this
treatment is given when they are in clinical remission. It is
also of some efficacy in the management of patients with
refractory Hodgkin's disease and non-Hodgkin's lymphoma,
although its place here is at present experimental and needs
to be clarified. It is also being employed experimentally in the
management of patients with advanced carcinomas, but the
results to date are not at all encouraging: quite high initial
response rates are followed by early relapse, and this treatment causes considerable morbidity and mortality.

For tissue compatibility the ideal donor of bone marrow is
an identical twin, but this of course is extremely unusual. A
patient does however have a one in four chance of being found
HLA identical on tissue typing with any given sibling. There
is an extremely low chance of being HLA identical with
anyone who is not a sibling but about 30 per cent of patients
have a suitable sibling donor. ABO incompatibility is not a
contraindication to grafting, but the complication rate rises
dramatically when marrow from a non-HLA identical donor

is used. For patients with leukaemia the chance of success rises when there is a female donor for a female recipient, but falls when there is a female donor for a male recipient.

Marrow is harvested by needle aspiration from multiple sites (anterior and posterior iliac crests and sternum) under general anaesthesia. At least $2 \times 10^8$ nucleated cells per recipient kilogram weight must be collected (700–1,000 ml for an adult). It is infused intravenously into the recipient and the stem cells then settle in their usual domicile. Production of neutrophils becomes apparent after about 20 days and that of platelets and red blood cells from between four to six weeks after infusion.

Drugs used in high dosage prior to BMT include cyclophosphamide (with mesna to prevent urothelial toxicity), melphalan, busulphan, etoposide, BCNU and CCNU; sometimes combinations of drugs are used. Total body irradiation (TBI) is usually given as well, using either fractionated or single dose regimens. Although BMT circumvents marrow toxicity, the dosages of drugs and irradiation are limited by their toxicities to other tissues, notably the lungs, liver, gastrointestinal tract and central nervous system. When TBI is given in a single fraction, higher doses and dose rates carry a significant risk of radiation pneumonitis. Sterility occurs in most patients and cataract formation can occur in patients surviving beyond two years.

## Autologous transplantation

Although autologous BMT does not give rise to problems from graft rejection, potential problems arise from the effects of previous chemotherapy and/or radiotherapy on the ability of the marrow to re-establish successfully adequate haematopoiesis, from contamination of the marrow with neoplastic cells, and from the loss of a graft versus leukaemia effect (see section below on graft versus host disease).

Various techniques have been used to try to purge marrow *in vitro* of neoplastic cells before reinfusion. These techniques include monoclonal antibodies linked to the toxin ricin or to cytotoxic drugs, or used to target magnetic colloids or polystyrene beads containing magnetite to the tumour cells which can then be removed using a high magnetic field. Non-

immunological approaches to the destruction of residual neoplastic cells have included the use of cytotoxic drugs and
tumour necrosis factor. However, it is almost certainly not
necessary to remove completely all the neoplastic cells from
reinfused marrow and it is highly unlikely anyway that any of
the techniques currently in use can achieve this. No controlled study has yet demonstrated the superiority of purged over
non-purged marrow.

## Allograft transplantation

Here there is no risk of infusion of neoplastic cells or of already
damaged marrow, but the toxicity is substantially greater
than with autologous BMT. This is due partly to graft versus
host disease (GVHD) and partly to the susceptibility to infection arising from the slow establishment of effective B- and
T-lymphocyte function. In particular, pneumonitis is common
and carries a high mortality. Its aetiology is multifactorial but
includes CMV infection, GVHD and radiation damage. The
risk can be reduced by using CMV negative blood products
when both the donor and recipient are CMV negative, and
also by fractionating total body irradiation or by using a low
dose rate if a single fraction is used.

## Graft versus host disease

Acute GVHD develops in approximately 50 per cent of patients. It may be minimal, with only a slight skin rash, or
severe with potentially fatal involvement of the skin, liver or
gut. Chronic GVHD develops in approximately 20 per cent of
patients surviving beyond 100 days. Manifestations include
scleroderma-like skin disease, buccal mucositis, keratocon-
junctivitis, liver, lung and gut involvement, generalised wasting and marked susceptibility to infections. GVHD can be
reduced in incidence and severity by prophylactic treatment
of the recipient with methotrexate and/or cyclosporin (see
below), or by depleting the infused marrow of T-lymphocytes
*in vitro* using physical separation methods (soybean lectin
agglutination or counterflow centrifugation) or monoclonal
antibodies. However, T-cell depletion results in an increased
risk of graft rejection and some GVHD appears to be bene-

ficial in patients with leukaemia through a graft versus leukaemia effect: syngeneic transplantation is followed by a three-fold increase in the risk of leukaemic relapse compared with allogeneic transplantation. These anti-GVHD measures have therefore had little impact on overall survival.

Mild to moderate acute GVHD can be treated with steroids but it does not always respond. Other treatments include anti-thymocyte globulin (ATG) and approaches involving monoclonal antibodies reacting with T-cells. The established treatment for chronic GVHD is low dose steroids in combination with azathioprine: 80 per cent of patients respond but treatment may need to be continued for one or two years. However, recent evidence suggests that thalidomide may have a useful rôle.

## Cyclosporin

This is a polypeptide with potent immunosuppressive activity, particularly against T-lymphocytes. It is usually administered in an oral solution but an intravenous infusion is available for use (in lower dosage) when absorption might be impaired or the oral preparation is not tolerated. Blood levels should be monitored – trough concentrations should be 250–1,000 ng/ml (equivalent to serum concentration of 50–200 ng/ml). The unpleasant taste may be masked by diluting the drug in milk or a fruit juice immediately before ingestion. It can affect liver and renal function and both should therefore be monitored. The latter may possibly be ameliorated by nifedipine. Care should be taken when considering the use of other potentially nephrotoxic drugs. It can also cause diabetes due to a toxic effect on β-cells, and the urine should be monitored. Other side effects include nausea, vomiting, tremor and hypertrichosis.

## Supportive care

This is crucial to the chances of success. This treatment causes pancytopenia and severe susceptibility to infection (see chapters on haematological disturbances, immunosuppression and infections). Mucositis can be severe and these patients may require parenteral nutrition. All blood products should be irradiated (15 Gy) to prevent GVHD caused by blood-donor T-lymphocytes, and consideration should be given to the use of white-cell filtrated products to reduce the incidence of CMV infection, and to prophylaxis against herpes infections and pneumocystis.

# Other Agents

## Bacteria

Stimulation of non-specific endogenous immune responses has been tried with both BCG and *Corynebacterium parvum*. Many studies have shown no benefit but there have been a few trials which have been reported as showing increased survival from the administration of BCG to patients with acute leukaemia, lymphoma and some solid tumours. Intravesical BCG is undoubtedly effective in the management of superficial bladder carcinoma, probably more so than intravesical cytotoxic drugs. The instillation of inactivated *Corynebacterium parvum* can be efficacious in preventing recurrence of malignant effusions, as are other agents which cause inflammation and fibrinous reactions such as talc and tetracycline.

## Interferons

As well as inhibiting viral replication, the interferons also inhibit cellular proliferation, stimulate cellular differentiation, increase tumour cell surface antigenicity, and stimulate cell-mediated immune activity. There are three main types: alpha, normally produced by leucocytes; beta, normally produced by fibroblasts; and gamma, normally produced by lymphocytes. Recombinant DNA technology has made it possible to produce large amounts of pure interferon.

Alpha interferon is effective against hairy cell leukaemia and Kaposi's sarcoma associated with AIDS, although it has now been replaced by deoxycoformycin as the drug of choice for hairy cell leukaemia. There has also been evidence of efficacy against other neoplasms, including lymphomas, melanoma, mycosis fungoides, myeloma, renal cell carcinoma and carcinoid and pancreatic endocrine tumours. However, there is no conclusive evidence that the interferons by themselves have curative potential for any malignancy, and toxicity is troublesome.

## Levamisole

This is an anti-helminthic drug for which an immunostimulant action has been claimed. As with BCG, there have been some trials in which it appears to have produced a marginal improvement in survival, but others in which no significant benefit has been demonstrated.

## Monoclonal antibodies

The administration of monoclonal antibodies directed against tumour cell antigens is an attractive concept. Cell death following binding of antibody, however, depends on the mobilisation of endogenous immune mechanisms which are unlikely to be sufficiently powerful to destroy very large numbers of tumour cells, and there has been little evidence of useful clinical efficacy. However, there have been reports of complete clinical responses in a small number of patients treated with monoclonal antibodies alone for non-Hodgkin's lymphoma and it is probable that anti-tumour effects can be enhanced if other agents acting as 'warheads' are bound to the monoclonal antibody, which is then used principally as a targeting mechanism. Such 'warheads' could include cytotoxic drugs, biological toxins and radioisotopes.

The clinical use of monoclonal antibodies for treatment at present is entirely experimental and there are several problems. The antigens present on tumour cells are invariably present on at least some of the normal cells as well. Human tumours are heterogeneous populations of cells and it is most unlikely that any particular antigen will be present on all the malignant cells. In addition, cell surface antigens often disappear quite rapidly after exposure to the antibody. Nevertheless, β-emitting radioisotopes can have a lethal range a couple of hundred cells away from the emitting atom and so the monoclonal antibody need not necessarily be linked to every malignant cell. Problems do however remain in delivering adequate amounts of antibody, and hence adequate irradiation, to malignant tissue; monoclonal antibody molecules are large and do not easily penetrate capillary basement membranes. A theoretical problem is the development of a human anti-mouse immune response with repeated administration. Cleaved antibodies (smaller fragments which retain their binding capacity) and 'humanised antibodies' are now both under evaluation.

## Retinoids

Retinoids control epithelial cell proliferation and differentiation. In animals they have been shown to prevent the development of frank neoplasia from pre-malignant conditions. Patients with cancer have been found to have lower serum retinoid levels than healthy controls, but recent evidence suggests that this is a consequence, rather than a cause, of their disease. Although there has been considerable interest in the possible rôle of retinoids in the management and possible prevention of human malignancy, their clinical use remains experimental, toxicity being one major problem. Retinoids have however been demonstrated to have some efficacy against mycosis fungoides, keratoacanthoma, multiple basal cell carcinomas, choriocarcinoma, squamous carcinomas of head, neck and lung, and in reducing the recurrence rate of superficial bladder cancer.

## NOTES

# NOTES

# CHAPTER 8

# Psychological Support

This is a very important part of the care of cancer patients but is all too frequently neglected because of lack of realisation and shortage of time. There is now an increasing number of voluntary organisations and groups which can often provide valuable support to patients, but this does not diminish the obligation of doctors to become involved as they are often able to provide valuable help in addition to counselling.

## Hidden concerns

Doctors tend to underestimate severely the need patients feel for discussing widely varying aspects of their disease, its treatment, and its impact on their lives, family and social relationships. Many patients do not feel free to discuss these matters with close relatives or friends and may feel lonely and isolated; both anxiety and depression are far more common than is usually apparent in busy clinical practice.

Most doctors develop techniques for the avoidance of discussion of matters which do not seem directly pertinent to the particular physical problem concerned, instead of taking the initiative and asking patients directly about how they feel in themselves. They do not ask about their reaction to the diagnosis and treatment, about how far their lives have otherwise returned to normal, about their body image and love-making, and indeed tend to ignore the cues, both verbal and non-verbal, that indicate that all is not quite as well as it may seem on the surface. Only a minority of patients will openly initiate discussion on psychosocial matters, whilst the remainder perhaps feel that the doctor's job is to be concerned only with physical aspects, that he is too busy or that they may appear to be ungrateful; indeed the subject may seem rather embarrassing to the patient.

## Specific problems

Patients with cancer have to come to terms with having an illness which could recur and kill them. Some have a severely altered body image as a result of mastectomy, laryngectomy, colostomy or other mutilation. They may feel that they have lost all attractiveness and they often lose libido and potency. They may not want to look at themselves naked in the mirror nor let their spouses see them naked or share a bed with them. Complete or marked loss of libido occurs in about one third of women after mastectomy.

Very commonly patients are reminded about their disease and vulnerability every time they have even the slightest symptom, attend for follow-up, or hear of the death from cancer of someone they know or of someone who is a well-known figure. In addition they may have other, sometimes irrational, worries. They may feel guilt from believing that they have brought the disease upon themselves as a result of smoking or as a result of being of a certain emotional disposition or having a particular lifestyle, and they may worry that the disease is infectious. They may feel a marked stigma and so withdraw from social life. In turn their families and friends often find it difficult to ask them how they are and thus seek to avoid discussion and even contact, and this can further increase a sense of isolation. Some tend to devalue their own doctor because he seems not to know as much about their illness as the doctor(s) in the cancer centre, and as a result they may be more reluctant to discuss their feelings with him than they would have done under other circumstances.

## Anxiety and depression

It has been found that as many as 25 per cent of cancer patients have either a clinically significant reactive depression, or an anxiety state which is substantially more profound than their previous normal and transient, adverse swings in mood. The incidence is usually somewhat higher in patients receiving particularly toxic treatment, younger patients, and in those with a poor prognosis, social problems and past psychiatric history.

These complications are usually persistent and accompanied by characteristic symptoms which may include anorexia, sleep disturbance, lack of concentration, memory impairment, irritability, feelings of guilt, hopelessness and pointlessness of life, suicidal feelings, persistent uncontrollable anxiety, panic attacks, sweating, palpitations and tremor. Some of these symptoms are present in up to 50 per cent of apparently tumour-free patients a whole year after the completion of potentially curative cytotoxic chemotherapy, although less than a quarter of these patients are usually diagnosed.

Those that are diagnosed are usually those that volunteer or demonstrate their psychological morbidity clearly in the ward, clinic or surgery. Some of these have obvious difficulty in coping with continued treatment, particularly cytotoxic chemotherapy. They can become increasingly more anxious and tense prior to each course, not necessarily because the physical side effects are difficult to cope with, but often because it is an unpleasant reminder of their disease and dependency on treatment. Some develop conditioned responses such as nausea and vomiting prior to drug administration and sometimes even on being reminded of any aspect of their treatment.

Psychiatric morbidity is more common in those patients who undergo additional treatment with cytotoxic chemotherapy after primary surgery. Cytotoxic chemotherapy may contribute to psychiatric toxicity through a direct chemical effect on the brain.

The importance of psychiatric diagnosis to the patient is that there is much that can be done to improve their symptoms, their quality of life and that of their families. Diagnosis depends on being aware of the significant chance of psychological morbidity in every cancer patient, of being sensitive and responsive to cues from patients, and on taking the initiative by asking relevant questions.

## Drug treatment

Reactive depression should not be dismissed as being understandable or a normal response in the circumstances. Treatment with tricyclic or tetracyclic drugs will help the great majority of patients; the latter drugs, for example mianserin, tend to be better tolerated. Perhaps just as important as drug treatment for many patients is the therapeutic benefit gained from being able to talk about their problems in the knowledge that someone understands. Patients with anxiety states will nearly always improve after the prescription of a benzodiazepine or phenothiazine tranquilliser; long-term administration is rarely necessary.

## Other approaches

Other psychological techniques can be helpful. These include demonstrating to patients that it is possible to challenge negative thoughts, relaxation exercises, positive imaging and desensitisation techniques where there is a problem with body image. There are also specialised psychosexual techniques which may be helpful where there is loss of libido. Many patients may benefit from referral to a psychiatrist or suitably experienced clinical psychologist.

**NOTES**

# NOTES

# CHAPTER 9

# Pain Control

The commonest causes of pain in patients with cancer are metastatic bone disease and nerve compression. However, it is important not to overlook non-malignant causes. In particular, degenerative bone and joint disease is common in the older age groups where cancer is most prevalent. It is also very important not to overlook pain control whilst waiting for anti-cancer-treatments to work.

### Anti-cancer treatments

Palliative radiotherapy is usually highly effective in controlling localised bone pain, often within a few days. Prolonged treatments are not necessary and usually only one fraction is required. Patients with widespread bone pain from multiple metastases, particularly from carcinoma of the prostate, may benefit considerably from double hemibody irradiation. Here single large radiation fractions (with prophylactic anti-emesis) are given to each half of the body, separated by usually 4–6 weeks to allow marrow recovery. Radiotherapy is also often effective in controlling pain arising from compression due to large visceral masses, although here treatment usually needs to be somewhat more prolonged.

Many patients will achieve pain relief from systemic treatment of their malignancy with hormonal or cytotoxic drugs, but usually this takes a little longer. Rapid improvement in bone pain is however sometimes seen following orchidectomy for metatatic prostate cancer, and following the now rarely performed hypophysectomy for patients with metastatic breast or prostate cancer.

## Analgesic drugs

### General

Analgesic drug therapy should be kept simple. It is best to gain experience with, and use only, a small number of agents. Pain can be well controlled with drugs in the majority of patients, usually using one of only three or four analgesic drugs. Most cancer pain is chronic and it is therefore essential that analgesics are taken regularly and not on a PRN basis: it is usually easier to prevent pain than to make it go away when it is already present. It is also essential that the drug given is of adequate potency and that it is given in an adequate dose.

The prevention of pain reduces anxiety which can often lower the pain threshold. For some patients diazepam or chlorpromazine may therefore be useful additions to the armamentarium. Depression can also lower the pain threshold and in some patients tricyclic, and related antidepressants, can help to control pain, as can other ways of improving morale.

### Milder analgesics

For milder pain paracetamol, by itself or in the slightly more effective combination with dextropropoxyphene (coproxamol), is usually effective and should be given four to six hourly. Dextropropoxyphene is a weak synthetic opioid but constipation is not usually troublesome. Another option for mild to moderate pain is dihydrocodeine. This has a greater tendency to cause constipation but it is available in a slow-release form which can be given 12-hourly. This can be helpful in improving pain control through the night, and compliance.

### Stronger analgesics

For more severe pain it is usually appropriate to proceed immediately to morphine or diamorphine elixir three to four hourly, or to slow-release morphine tablets. The usual required dose range for oral morphine is 5–200 mg 3–4 hourly, but 90 per cent of cancer patients do not require more than

30 mg doses. Morphine is now available in a concentrated oral solution which is particularly useful for patients on high doses: it can conveniently be added to a soft drink. It is also available in a slow-release form which is more convenient for many patients, and particularly helpful in achieving pain control throughout the night. This is usually taken 12-hourly and never needs to be taken more frequently than 8-hourly. For most patients there is thus little point in starting with less than 30 mg doses. The appropriate dose of morphine is the dose required to alleviate the pain. The dose should be increased, rather than the frequency of administration, usually in preference to taking another weaker analgesic between doses. There is no problem of addiction in patients with incurable cancer. There is no maximum dose.

There is no special advantage in giving diamorphine instead of morphine for oral administration, but it is more suitable for parenteral use because of greater solubility. Buprenorphine is sometimes considered an attractive narcotic analgesic for cancer pain. It is given sublingually and has a duration of action lasting 8–12 hours. However, its absorption may be particularly unreliable in patients who have a dry mouth. It must also be remembered that, like pentazocine (which is a poor analgesic for cancer patients), it has narcotic antagonist as well as agonist properties. It should therefore not be given concurrently with morphine or diamorphine and some patients may experience transiently increased pain when it is substituted by morphine or diamorphine. Buprenorphine in a dose of 0.2 mg 8 hourly is approximately equivalent to 10–15 mg of morphine 4 hourly.

Anti-emetics may need to be given initially with opiates but nausea from these drugs nearly always fades away after a few days. Drowsiness too nearly always subsides, although it may return transiently with dose escalation. However, constipation persists and is exacerbated by poor dietary and fluid intake and reduced mobility. It is wise to prescribe routinely the regular administration of a laxative, for example lactulose, for these patients. They should also be encouraged to have a good intake of fluid, fruit, green vegetables and fibre.

### Rectal administration

Morphine suppositories may be helpful where swallowing is difficult, or oral drugs poorly tolerated because of nausea, vomiting, weakness or drowsiness. The dosage should be the same as for oral administration.

### Parenteral administration

This is necessary for some patients, at least initially. Diamorphine is preferable to morphine because it is more soluble. When changing from oral morphine to parenteral diamorphine the dose should initially be divided by 3, and by 2 when changing from oral diamorphine, because of the increased bioavailability. Patients who require regular injections may benefit from a continuous slow subcutaneous infusion into the anterior abdominal wall via a butterfly needle, using a syringe driver; the needle needs to be resited every three days or so. A day's supply of diamorphine can be dissolved in 5–10 ml of sterile water – saline should not be used.

### Other drugs

Patients with bone pain often benefit from the addition of a non-steroidal anti-inflammatory drug such as aspirin 600–1200 mg 4 hourly, or naproxen. Such drugs should be taken with food or milk. Suppositories are available, which may improve gastro-intestinal tolerance.

Pain from nerve compression or infiltration is sometimes helped by the addition of the membrane-stabilising anti-arrhythmic drug flecainide in a dose of 100 mg bd. It is usually reasonably well tolerated although dizziness and visual disturbances can occur. However, it can occasionally promote severe arrhythmias and there is evidence that patients given this drug following myocardial infarction experience a slight absolute increase in the risk of death. It should therefore be considered only in patients with advanced disease. Other drugs worth considering for this type of pain include carbamazepine (100 mg tds), sodium valproate (200 mg tds) or clonazepam (0.5–2.0 mg once/twice daily). The muscle relaxant baclofen may help when a component of pain is due to increased muscle tone or spasm. Alternatively diazepam may be used, but it is more sedative.

Anti-osteoclast medication with a calcitonin infusion or short course of diphosphonate can benefit some patients with widespread bone pain that is otherwise difficult to control (see section on hypercalcaemia).

## Pain relief clinic

### Nerve blocks

In a minority of patients, pain cannot be satisfactorily controlled with medication. They may benefit from referral to a pain clinic, usually run by a consultant anaesthetist, for consideration of a nerve block. A variety of interventions is available, depending on the site of pain. The infiltration is usually initially with local anaesthetic and/or steroid, in which case the effect is usually transient. Surprisingly, however, benefit is often achieved for several weeks. Some patients may be deemed suitable for a permanent (neurolytic) nerve block, usually achieved by injecting phenol. Nerve blocks are often given into the epidural or intrathecal space, but neurolytic blocks are usually considered only if the pain is unilateral and limited to a few dermatomes, for fear of damaging sphincter control or causing paresis. Patients with pancreatic and other abdominal pain often benefit from a coeliac plexus block and those with chest wall pain from an intercostal nerve block.

### Epidural diamorphine infusion

Continuous infusion of diamorphine into the epidural space is sometimes used for patients with severe lumbosacral pain and can be highly effective over long periods. Relatively small doses may be sufficient, thereby lessening systemic side effects.

### Transcutaneous electric nerve stimulation

This is a safe non-invasive method of obtaining transient pain relief which has been used successfully in some patients with localised, but usually less severe, pain.

## Neurosurgery

Very occasionally patients with a relatively good prognosis will be considered for neurosurgical procedures such as cutting of the dorsal sensory roots for the affected dermatomes, or a cordotomy, when the spinothalamic tract within the spinal cord is interrupted in the cervical or thoracic region. About 90 per cent of patients experience good pain relief initially following cordotomy, but this procedure carries a ≤5 per cent risk of severe neurological complications and some degree of pain returns in about half the patients during the subsequent twelve months.

**NOTES**

# NOTES

# CHAPTER 10

# Other Symptom Causes and Control

### Anorexia

This is a very common symptom, particularly in patients with advanced disease. In addition to anorexia *per se*, taste perversions and food aversions are also very common, both before and after treatment with radiotherapy or chemotherapy. They are reminiscent of those occurring in pregnancy and it is interesting that women with cancer quite often develop the same aversions they experienced many years earlier during pregnancy. Seasoning and a readiness to try alternatives can sometimes help.

Small meals at frequent intervals are often more acceptable than larger meals at conventional times. They should be attractively prepared and a glass of sherry before a meal can sometimes stimulate appetite. Steroids, e.g. prednisolone 15–20 mg daily, are often useful in the stimulation of appetite in patients with advanced disease. Progestogens in high dosage can also increase the appetite and weight of some patients, without the fluid retention and other side effects normally associated with prednisolone or dexamethasone. (See section on malnutrition.)

It has been reported that exposing the patient to a 'scapegoat' nutritionally inconsequential food, such as a fruit-flavoured drink, immediately prior to a first course of chemotherapy can result in 'targeting' of any food aversion against that particular flavour, thereby sparing acceptable and desirable items in the patient's normal diet.

## Anxiety

See chapter on psychological support.

## Confusion

The commonest cause of confusion in young and middle-aged cancer patients is brain metastases, often presenting as a subtle personality change or persistent headache. This is also a common cause in the elderly, but this age group is prone to develop confusion from other causes such as toxicity from treatments directed against their malignancies, other medication (e.g. opiates, steroids), infection and change of environment, particularly hospitalisation. Confusion can also be caused by electrolyte disturbances (hypercalcaemia and hyponatraemia), hyper- and hypo-glycaemia, hypoxia, liver failure, non-neoplastic encephalopathies (para-neoplastic, viral and methotrexate-induced) and hyper-viscosity. (See specific sections.) Where possible and appropriate the underlying cause should be treated, but it is often necessary to reassure the relatives, and sometimes the patient.

## Constipation

This extremely common complaint in cancer patients is usually due to any or all of poor dietary intake (including lack of roughage), analgesics and immobility. Other causes include dehydration, hypercalcaemia, obstruction due to intrinsic or extrinsic tumour, and spinal cord or cauda equina pathology. The cytotoxic vinca alkaloids (particularly vincristine) cause autonomic neuropathy. Rarely, intestinal obstruction is due to a radiation stricture. Constipation may present with spurious diarrhoea because of impaction with overflow.

### Laxatives

For many patients regular administration of laxatives is necessary, particularly those receiving opiate drugs (e.g. lactulose 15 ml bd, which is usually effective and not unpleasant to taste). In terminal care a faecal softener combined with a peristaltic stimulant is useful. Bulk-forming agents are helpful in the management of patients with an ileostomy or colostomy. It is important to ensure that patients taking these drugs have an adequate fluid intake to avoid obstruction due to faecal impaction. Lactulose is particularly effective for constipation due to vincristine. Great caution should be taken in prescribing laxatives, particularly stimulant laxatives, where there is the possibility of bowel obstruction.

## Obstruction

Although surgical intervention is appropriate for many patients with bowel obstruction, patients with terminal disease and bowel obstruction can usually be saved from surgery with skilled medical management. (See specific section.)

## Cough

Causes of cough of particular relevance to cancer patients are primary and secondary lung tumours, infection, and pneumonitis caused by radiation or cytotoxic drugs. For patients with pulmonary neoplasia usually only those with primary bronchial carcinoma are likely to derive significant symptomatic benefit from palliative radiotherapy. However, mediastinal lymphadenopathy (e.g. from breast carcinoma) often responds well to radiotherapy.

Non-opiate cough suppressants are rarely useful. However, methadone, morphine and diamorphine can be very effective in suppressing distressing cough in patients with advanced lung cancer. Subcutaneous hyoscine can be helpful where secretions are excessive. Steroids can be of substantial benefit in patients with lymphangitis carcinomatosa or radiation pneumonitis. (See section on dyspnoea.) In some patients coughing is aggravated in certain positions and practical advice about avoiding such positions can be helpful, e.g. sleeping in a chair.

## Depression

See chapter on psychological support.

## Diarrhoea

Causes include neoplastic involvement of bowel, spurious diarrhoea, radiotherapy, some cytotoxic drugs (e.g. methotrexate, 5-fluorouracil), antibiotics, ileostomy and colostomy, post-gastrectomy syndrome and paraneoplastic humoral activity (e.g. carcinoid syndrome, medullary thyroid carcinoma). It is occasionally caused by an excessive intake of fruit and raw vegetables in patients on 'alternative' diets.

Abdominal or pelvic radiotherapy frequently causes diarrhoea. This usually comes on a couple of weeks after the start of treatment, but sometimes sooner. Codeine phosphate, kaolin and morphine mixture, diphenoxylate and loperamide are all useful. It is important to maintain a good fluid intake, and it is sometimes necessary for there to be a break in the course of treatment, particularly when there is associated abdominal pain and peritonism. Methylcellulose is useful in patients with an ileostomy or colostomy.

## Dysphagia

This is most commonly caused by malignant tumours of the upper aero-digestive tract. Some patients are eligible for potentially curative treatment but the majority have incurable tumours and for these only palliation is feasible. Obstruction due to tumour characteristically causes dysphagia which is worse for solids than liquids. This is reversed in the minority of patients whose dysphagia is due to neuromuscular deficiency. This may be due to conditions such as bulbar palsy or myasthenia, but infiltration by advanced tumours can also interfere with normal neuromuscular function.

External radiotherapy is moderately effective in relieving dysphagia due to intrinsic or extrinsic carcinoma. Intracavitary radiotherapy using a remote afterloading machine is now a feasible, quick and usually effective palliative treatment for patients with oesophageal carcinoma. For the rare patients whose dysphagia is due to Hodgkin's disease or non-Hodgkin's lymphoma cytotoxic chemotherapy or radiotherapy will usually provide rapid relief.

For many of these patients however, palliation is most quickly achieved with endoscopic intubation. This is usually well tolerated but it is not technically feasible for all patients and there is a risk of perforation. The risks of morbidity and mortality from this procedure are greater in frail patients, and those who are terminally ill may be more appropriately managed by conservative methods. This may include attention to food consistency, hydration, pain control, treatment of any candidiasis, anti-emesis and alternative routes for medication (rectally, subcutaneously or intravenously).

## Dyspnoea

Possible causes of particular relevance in cancer patients include anaemia, primary or secondary lung tumour, pleural or pericardial effusion or fibrosis, ascites, tumour in a major airway, lung infection, pneumothorax due to peripheral tumour and pulmonary embolism. Iatrogenic causes include radiation pneumonitis, cytotoxic drug pneumonitis or fibrosis and pneumothorax after pleural aspiration.

In terminally ill patients the distress associated with dyspnoea from any cause may be substantially alleviated by opiates and diazepam. In these patients opiates should not be withheld because of the fear that they may produce respiratory depression.

### Stridor

A tracheostomy may be lifesaving for patients with stridor from tumour obstructing the larynx or higher, as may urgent radiotherapy for obstruction a little lower down. Steroids (e.g. dexamethasone 4 mg tds for a few days only) are usually given in addition to radiotherapy, with the aim of lessening any oedematous component in or around the tumour, or any oedema arising as a result of radiotherapy. Laser treatment can also be used to debulk tumour within a major airway.

### Lymphangitis carcinomatosa

Patients with pulmonary lymphangitis carcinomatosa (most commonly seen in metastatic breast carcinoma) may experience severe dyspnoea, sometimes with cough, but often have few other clinical signs. The chest X-ray may also look remarkably normal at first, although later widespread linear opacification is usually seen. The symptoms are often rapidly relieved by steroids, e.g. prednisolone 10 mg tds reducing to 5 mg tds after a few days.

## Pleural effusion

This is the commonest cause of dyspnoea in cancer patients. Effusions are seen most commonly in patients with breast, bronchial and ovarian carcinoma. Cytological examination of the fluid does not always reveal malignant cells but the fluid is almost always an exudate. Repeated re-accumulation of fluid may warrant a pleurodesis, which is usually effective in preventing significant recurrence in about two-thirds of patients. (See specific section.)

## Opportunistic lung infection

This can occur in immunosuppressed patients, particularly patients with leukaemia and lymphoma and those who are treated aggressively. Pulmonary infection with *Pneumocystis carinii* can cause severe respiratory insufficiency and dry cough with remarkably clear auscultation. Other opportunistic causes of lung infection include cytomegalovirus, herpes zoster, aspergillus and tuberculosis. (See chapter on immunosuppression and infections.)

## Radiation pneumonitis

This causes a dry cough, sometimes with dyspnoea. It becomes apparent a month or two after radiotherapy and may be provoked by chest infection. Although the risk of pneumonitis is dependent on the volume of lung irradiated and the dose given, it can occur whenever a moderate amount of lung tissue is irradiated to even quite modest doses. It is well recognised following radiotherapy for breast carcinoma, when some lung irradiation is usually inevitable: parenchymal opacification may be seen on the chest X-ray, usually situated in the upper zone and anteriorly. Pneumonitis is reversible, but some degree of permanent fibrosis is usual, although rarely severe. Far more severe and potentially fatal bilateral pneumonitis can sometimes occur after high dose whole or upper body irradiation.

The acute symptoms are often rapidly improved by steroids, e.g. prednisolone 20–30 mg daily. However steroids are of no value in fibrosis, and will not prevent its development.

## Cytotoxic drug pneumonitis

Several cytotoxic drugs can cause pneumonitis and pulmonary fibrosis, especially bleomycin and busulphan. Steroids again may improve the acute symptoms. Chemotherapy can act synergistically with radiotherapy to produce more severe lung toxicity.

## Pericardial effusion

This can be caused by tumour invasion or high dose irradiation. It characteristically causes right heart failure, faint heart sounds and pulsation, and a 'pulsus paradoxus'. This is not really paradoxical, merely an exaggeration of the normal fall in systolic pressure during inspiration. It is considered present if the fall is >10 mm Hg. A pericardial rub is often heard and the chest X-ray usually arouses suspicion by showing an enlarged and rounded heart shadow. The diagnosis is easily confirmed by ultrasound. There is usually rapid relief of dyspnoea following aspiration. Repeated re-accumulation can be an indication for surgery with the creation of a pericardial 'window' in selected patients. Other options include irradiation (when neoplasia is the cause) and the instillation of tetracycline or cytotoxic drugs into the pericardial sac. These last options may however predispose towards subsequent pericardial fibrosis.

## Fever

Malignant disease can by itself cause fever, e.g. Hodgkin's disease and renal carcinoma, but until there is very good evidence to the contrary it should be presumed that fever is due to infection. The possibility of infection in any immunosuppressed patient should be taken especially seriously.

Lymphoproliferative malignancies, leukaemias and their

treatments can be particularly immunosuppressive, but any patient receiving cytotoxic chemotherapy may become susceptible to infection as a result of leucopenia. Septicaemia is a common event in severely leucopenic patients and should be treated very promptly. (See chapter on immunosuppression and infections.)

Fever caused directly by tumour may be suppressed with steroids. Some cytotoxic drugs (e.g. bleomycin) can produce a febrile reaction.

## Haemorrhage

### Tumour

Radiotherapy is usually highly effective in controlling bleeding from tumours at any site, but usually takes a few days to work. Where haemorrhage is very heavy other measures may need to be considered, depending principally on the site. These may include diathermy or cryosurgery, excision, packing, arterial embolisation or ligation.

### Thrombocytopenia

Although haemorrhage frequently occurs from cancers in a variety of different sites it is important to remember that some patients may have a haemorrhagic tendency, most commonly due to thrombocytopenia. This is usually apparent as a result of bleeding occurring at sites where there is no tumour, e.g. purpura or epistaxis. The fundi should be examined since retinal haemorrhage is an indication for platelet transfusion. Thrombocytopenia may be caused by the disease itself (marrow infiltration, hypersplenism) or by marrow suppression as a result of treatment (cytotoxic chemotherapy, systemic irradiation). (See specific section.)

### Disseminated intravascular coagulation

This less common cause of a haemorrhagic tendency may involve massive consumption and depletion of clotting factors and platelets. It can occur as a direct complication of advanced malignancy, particularly carcinomas of pancreas and prostate and acute leukaemia, as well as septicaemia. (See specific section.)

## Radiation telangiectasia

This is usually seen only after high dose (radical) radiotherapy. The sites usually involved are the bladder, rectum and vagina. Radiation proctitis often responds well to steroid enemas or suppositories. Gentle diathermy can be effective at any site, particularly if the source is relatively localised, but excessive diathermy may worsen haemorrhage by causing an indolent ulcer.

For patients with troublesome bleeding from bladder telangiectasia other possible measures include hydrostatic bladder distension, and the instillation of formalin into the bladder under general anaesthesia and with very strict precautions. 500–1000 ml of formalin solution (1 per cent or higher if necessary, but not >10 per cent) is retained in the bladder for 10–30 minutes. A cystogram must be performed prior to the procedure to exclude vesico-ureteric reflux, and the pressure must not exceed 15 cms; the bladder must subsequently be washed out with distilled water. This technique is often successful in controlling bleeding. Other intravesical solutions which may be tried include silver nitrate and alum.

Anti-fibrinolytic drugs (tranexamic acid, aminocaproic acid) are sometimes useful in the short-term management of haemorrhage. They should be avoided if there is a previous history of thrombo-embolic disease and they may result in clot retention in patients with urinary tract bleeding.

## Headache

Headache due to intracranial tumour, primary or secondary, is characteristically worse on waking in the morning. The raised intracranial pressure may be lowered by a reduction in cerebral oedema. Dexamethasone, initially in divided dosage of 8–16 mg daily, is often highly effective in improving headache and other associated symptoms; in many patients the dose can later be reduced to 4 mg daily. Other neoplastic causes to consider are skull and cervical spine metastases and hyperviscosity. (See section on brain metastases.)

## Malaise

For patients with advanced cancer, and when it is concluded that malaise is attributable to nothing other than the malignancy, considerable improvement may result from steroids, e.g. prednisolone 20–30 mg daily.

## Malodour

Fungating tumours are often colonised with anaerobic organisms. Metronidazole 400 mg tds for 5–7 days will often improve the unpleasant smell. This drug can cause alcohol intolerance.

## Nausea and vomiting

Causes include cytotoxic chemotherapy, radiotherapy, advanced tumour, liver metastases, hypercalcaemia, hyponatraemia, intestinal obstruction, brain metastases and opiates.

In addition to the variety of available specific anti-emetic drugs some patients will experience significant benefit from steroids, e.g. prednisolone 15–30 mg daily or dexamethasone 2–4 mg daily. However, their continuous use for this indication is only appropriate for patients with terminal disease. Prochlorperazine and domperidone are available as suppositories. Metoclopramide should not be prescribed in patients with intestinal obstruction as it increases small bowel motility.

### Cytotoxic chemotherapy

The nausea and vomiting from chemotherapy is quite often unpredictable, although some drugs, e.g. cisplatin and DTIC, will cause it almost universally. Psychological factors can be important and this side effect can become progressively more severe with each course of treatment. It can become a conditioned response and may even become an anticipatory phenomenon, occurring before drug administration. It may also return long after treatment has finished when the patient goes back to hospital or even drives past it or sees his oncologist. The timing and duration is very variable. It may start immediately after the injection, but more commonly after several (often 10–12) hours. It may be very transient, last only a few hours, or extend over several days or even weeks. Some patients describe persisting though often intermittent nausea from one course to the next. For many patients nausea is a far more unpleasant phenomenon than vomiting.

For patients receiving drug regimens known to have a high chance of causing severe nausea and vomiting prophylactic anti-emesis is essential. Prophylaxis is also advisable for the great majority of patients receiving other regimens and successful prevention at the start of a course of treatment may help to prevent a subsequent conditioned response. It has been demonstrated that 24-hour pre-treatment with anti-emetics (domperidone and dexamethasone) significantly reduces nausea and vomiting compared with starting anti-emetics at the time of administration of chemotherapy. Some patients benefit from benzodiazepine tranquillisers taken orally two to three days prior to treatment.

Ideally anti-emetics should be given parenterally at the time of the cytotoxic injection, and subsequently in patients receiving highly emetic treatments. However for many patients, particularly those receiving treatment as out-patients, oral administration is effective and sufficient, although some will find suppositories very helpful. It is often helpful to administer anti-emetics regularly, rather than on a PRN basis, over the day or days immediately following injection. Patients should be advised not to drive immediately after receiving chemotherapy and anti-emetics.

A minority of patients develop apparently intractable severe nausea and vomiting which is unresponsive to standard measures. If continued treatment is considered essential major sedation (e.g. with high dosage lorazepam) may be required. Some success has been reported using hypnosis and acupuncture. For patients with severe vomiting attention to fluid balance is important.

Drugs commonly used 4–8 hourly for chemotherapy nausea and vomiting include the following:

Dexamethasone    8 mg IV/IM stat. then 2–4 mg PO/IM/IV. It is often useful to combine dexamethasone with another anti-emetic.

| | |
|---|---|
| Domperidone | 10–20 mg PO; 60 mg PR. |
| Lorazepam | 1–2 mg IV; 1–2.5 mg PO. Prolonged use should be avoided due to risk of dependence. |
| Metoclopramide (low dose) | 10–20 mg IV stat then PO/IV. Low dose metoclopramide is rather less effective than dexamethasone or domperidone. |
| Metoclopramide (high dose) | Maximum of 10 mg/kg over 24 hours in IV infusion. Continuous infusion is more effective than intermittent infusion of the same total dose. In-patient administration only. It is compatible with cisplatin, cyclophosphamide and adriamycin but should not be mixed with other cytotoxic drugs. Extrapyramidal reactions occur in under 10 per cent of patients overall but are more common in younger and elderly debilitated patients: parenteral orphenadrine, benztropine or procyclidine may be required.<br><br>Metoclopramide can precipitate acute hypertension in patients with phaeochromocytoma. |
| Nabilone | 1–2 mg PO bd. May be usefully started the evening before treatment. Drowsiness and other CNS side effects are quite common; euphoria and hallucinations may be reduced or prevented with concurrent phenothiazine administration. |
| Prochlorperazine | 12.5 mg IV/IM stat. then 10 mg PO or 25 mg PR. Extrapyramidal reactions occur only very occasionally in younger and elderly debilitated patients. |

## Paresis/paralysis

See section on spinal cord/cauda equina compression.

## Pruritus

Cholestyramine can relieve the itching of obstructive jaundice where the biliary obstruction is only partial. It acts by sequestering bile acids and is contra-indicated when biliary obstruction is complete. There is then no gut absorption of bilirubin and therefore no urobilinogen in the urine. This drug is unfortunately unpleasant to take and often causes nausea and diarrhoea.

Cimetidine is sometimes helpful in controlling the pruritus of Hodgkin's disease but this usually responds rapidly to effective oncological treatment. Cimetidine, antihistamines and topical sodium cromoglycate have all had some effectiveness against the pruritus of polycythaemia. Other measures which are sometimes helpful include steroids and crotamiton or local anaesthetic creams.

## Stomatitis/oesophagitis

Neoplastic involvement of the mouth and oesophagus will often cause soreness by itself. Other common causes are cytotoxic chemotherapy, local radiotherapy, iron and vitamin deficiency, and infection. Candidal infections are very common and usually rapidly respond to nystatin or amphotericin lozenges. In immunosuppressed patients herpes simplex infection is also a common cause and often clear-cut ulceration is not seen; a high index of suspicion is necessary since acyclovir can be rapidly effective. (See specific sections.)

Soreness from radiation mucositis or post-chemotherapy ulceration may be alleviated with aspirin gargles, salicylic dental gel, analgesic mouthwashes (e.g. benzydamine) and local anaesthetic (e.g. benzocaine) lozenges. Regular attention to oral hygiene with frequent cleansing mouthwashes is advisable. False teeth must be taken out prior to mouthwashes or topical anti-fungal treatment. Radiation oesophagitis is often relieved with Mucaine. When methotrexate is the cause of oral ulceration a calcium folinate mouthwash may be helpful.

## Weakness

Weakness is an almost inevitable aspect of very advanced disease but in patients who are not clearly terminally ill it is important to consider other causes, some of which may be treatable. These include anaemia, malnutrition, prolonged bed rest, leg oedema, paraneoplastic neuromyopathy, steroid myopathy, spinal cord or cauda equina compression, hypoadrenalism (adrenal or pituitary metastasis), hyponatraemia (a feature of paraneoplastic inappropriate ADH secretion) and hypokalaemia (seen with diarrhoea, steroids and diuretics, and excessive mineralocorticoid secretion due to ectopic tumour production of ACTH or adrenal cortical tumour). Some patients benefit from physiotherapy and encouragement to carry out exercises, on the bed if necessary. Postural hypotension is also a very common occurrence in patients with advanced cancer, secondary to an autonomic neuropathy which may possibly be caused by malnutrition or develop as a paraneoplastic phenomenon.

## NOTES

# NOTES

# CHAPTER 11

# Haematological Disturbances

Deficiency of all or any of the cellular constituents of blood is common in clinical oncology, frequently occurring with aggressive tumours and/or aggressive treatments. Potential causes of pancytopenia include cytotoxic chemotherapy, neoplastic infiltration of the bone marrow, hypersplenism and whole body or very extensive radiotherapy. Marrow infiltration is of course inevitable in leukaemia and multiple myeloma but it is also a very common occurrence in non-Hodgkin's lymphoma and to a lesser extent with some carcinomas, notably those of breast, bronchus and prostate. Marrow infiltration is often suggested by the appearance in the peripheral blood of immature red and white blood cells (leucoerythroblastic anaemia). Treatment of the causative malignancy may result in haematological recovery but for patients with carcinomatous marrow infiltration cytotoxic chemotherapy should be given very cautiously in an attempt to avoid a potentially hazardous severe worsening of the haematological disturbance prior to any subsequent response. Splenectomy may be performed for hypersplenism but low dose-rate splenic irradiation is less hazardous and is sometimes highly effective.

Meticulous monitoring of the blood count is essential in all patients receiving cytotoxic chemotherapy and wide-field radiotherapy. Trends, as well as absolute levels, should be taken into account when deciding whether or not to proceed with further treatment. Treatment directed against the causative malignancy and also that aimed at correcting the haematological disturbance are not always indicated. Many of these patients are entering the terminal phase of their illness, for which further active treatment has little or no chance of success, and repeated transfusions may serve only to prolong suffering and perhaps allow the patient to live long enough to experience new and more unpleasant symptoms than weakness.

Other causes for specific abnormalities, with notes on management, are now given:

## Anaemia

Other common causes include chronic disease *per se* (normochromic, normocytic), haemorrhage (hypochromic, microcytic), infection, impaired nutrition, haemolysis and disseminated intravascular coagulation (see separate sections). Transfusion is not always necessary, particularly if the anaemia is mild and asymptomatic, and not always appropriate (see above). There is evidence to suggest that peri-operative transfusion can impair the long-term prognosis (see chapter on surgery), but patients receiving radiotherapy should ideally have a haemoglobin concentration >12.0 g/dl in order to reduce radioresistance consequent on tumour cell hypoxia. For most patients packed cells are sufficient, but whole blood (when available, and preferably fresh) is helpful in massive haemorrhage where there is a requirement for volume and clotting factor replacement. Blood transfusion can precipitate potentially fatal haemorrhage in patients who are already seriously thrombocytopenic ($<30 \times 10^9$/litre) and those patients at risk should receive platelet cover.

## Disseminated intravascular coagulation (DIC)

Overt DIC occurs occasionally as a direct complication of advanced malignancy but more commonly as a complication of septicaemia, particularly in immunosuppressed patients. Although DIC can be an extremely acute and severe process carrying a very poor prognosis it occurs more commonly in a milder, chronic, subclinical form particularly in patients with advanced lung, prostate, breast and pancreatic cancer. DIC results in excessive consumption of platelets, clotting factors and red blood cells thereby leading to thrombocytopenia, haemorrhage and anaemia. There is an increased level in the blood of fibrin-fibrinogen degradation products (FDP) and these exert a further anticoagulant effect. Occlusion of small blood vessels can result in renal failure or brain damage.

Treatment of clinical DIC, if appropriate, requires vigorous attention to the underlying cause and replacement of haemostatic factors with the use of fresh frozen plasma and platelet transfusions. The use of heparin to block the coagulation process remains controversial: it can be very hazardous but should be considered when thrombosis is thought to be responsible for organ damage (e.g. 15,000–25,000 units/24 hours). Oral anticoagulants are usually ineffective. The use of antifibrinolytic agents is also controversial but these should be considered when there is laboratory evidence that fibrinolysis is a major component, e.g. aprotinin 500,000 kallidinogenase inactivator units by slow intravenous injection followed by 200,000 units via intravenous infusion every 4 hours; tranexamic acid 3–6 g daily orally or 3 g daily by slow intravenous injection in divided doses. Simultaneous administration of heparin is probably advisable with these drugs.

## Graft versus host disease (GVHD)

This occurs most commonly after bone marrow transplantation (see section in chapter on drug treatment) although transfusion of blood products can cause acute GVHD in patients with severely impaired cell-mediated immunity, especially those with Hodgkin's disease and acute leukaemia. This may become apparent 4–30 days after transfusion and the clinical features include pancytopenia, generalised erythroderma and liver and gastrointestinal toxicity. Although rare, this syndrome is at present underdiagnosed. The skin biopsy appearances are characteristic but proof depends on the demonstration of circulating lymphocytes with a different HLA type from that of the host cells. Irradiation of blood products (15 Gy) is mandatory after bone marrow transplantation and has also been advocated for patients receiving intensive chemotherapy for advanced Hodgkin's disease or acute leukaemia.

## Hyperviscosity

Plasma hyperviscosity occurs most commonly in Waldenström's macroglobulinaemia and multiple myeloma. The high molecular weight of the IgM molecule results in symptomatic hyperviscosity [which usually occurs at levels of plasma viscosity >4 milli-Pascales (relative to water)] being far more common in patients with macroglobulinaemia (approximately 50 per cent) than myeloma (approximately 3 per cent).

Hyperviscosity causes a haemorrhagic tendency, retinopathy with haemorrhages and papilloedema, CNS symptoms and signs from weakness to coma, hypervolaemia and cardiac failure. Plasmapharesis is effective by removing the paraprotein: 4–6 units of plasma should be removed daily until the viscosity falls below 4, in conjunction with chemotherapy for the underlying neoplasm.

Hyperviscosity of whole blood may be caused not only by plasma hyperviscosity but also by substantial increases in cell counts, as in acute or chronic (usually myeloid) leukaemia and polycythaemia (rubra vera or secondary to other causes including renal carcinoma, hepatoma and other cancers). Very high white cell counts ($>100 \times 10^9$/litre) can result in intravascular leukaemic cell aggregation (leukostasis) in the brain, lungs and elsewhere with symptoms and signs similar to those from plasma hyperviscosity and carrying a risk of cerebral haemorrhage. In the acute situation the rapid destruction of intracerebral aggregates of leukaemic cells with immediate cranial irradiation, leukapharesis using blood cell separators, and venesection for polycythaemia can all be of substantial benefit. Blood transfusion in patients with high whole blood viscosity can result in a highly dangerous further increase.

## Leucopenia

The risk of infection only rises significantly when the neutrophil count falls below $1.0 \times 10^9$/litre. Cytotoxic chemotherapy impairs neutrophil function as well as reducing numbers. Corticosteroids also impair neutrophil function.

Transfusion of granulocytes is still controversial and only rarely undertaken, but should be considered in patients with severe neutropenia (count $<0.5 \times 10^9$/litre) and severe infection not responding to antibiotics after 24 hours, particularly if early bone marrow recovery is not anticipated. There is no indication for prophylactic administration. The best method of harvesting is with the use of a continuous-flow cell separator; the removal of the buffy coat from fresh whole blood usually provides only a poor yield. Granulocyte transfusions carry a risk of fever, sequestration in the pulmonary circulation and CMV infection.

Lithium carbonate can normally induce leucocytosis. The prophylactic administration of lithium carbonate in an initial dose of 300 mg tds (subsequently adjusted on the basis of weekly estimations with the aim of achieving a serum concentration in the normal psychiatric range of 0.6–1.2 mmol/litre) has been shown to reduce both neutropenia and the incidence of infection in patients receiving chemotherapy for carcinoma but not leukaemia. Side effects such as nausea, vomiting, weakness, drowsiness and giddiness are however quite common and justify a dose reduction. More severe CNS toxicity may require cessation of treatment.

Granulocyte colony stimulating factor (GCSF) can now be manufactured and early clinical experience indicates that it can both stimulate *in vivo* production of neutrophils and reduce the incidence of infection in patients receiving cytotoxic chemotherapy. However, there is also evidence suggesting that it can stimulate clonogenic leukaemic blast cells in patients with acute myeloid leukaemia.

## Thrombocytopenia

Other aetiologies include those causing increased peripheral destruction such as disseminated intravascular coagulation and chemotherapy with vinblastine, bleomycin and cisplatinum for germ cell tumours. Both haemorrhage and infection can also reduce platelet survival. Severe anaemia has been shown to increase the risk of haemorrhage in thrombocytopenia. However, blood transfusion lowers the platelet count and if this is already low ($<30 \times 10^9$/litre) serious complications can arise if platelet cover is not given. Normally spontaneous bleeding occurs only if the platelet count falls below $20 \times 10^9$/litre, but can occur at higher levels if the patient is pyrexial or taking anti-coagulants, aspirin, other non-steroidal anti-inflammatory drugs, alcohol, or high doses of penicillin or its analogues (e.g. carbenicillin, ticarcillin), since all these can impair platelet function. Even minor trauma must be avoided in these patients, including such measures as the use of electric razors and the avoidance of intramuscular or subcutaneous injections, hard or vigorous tooth-brushing, vigorous nose blowing, vigorous unlubricated sexual intercourse and straining at stool. Pressure should be applied to injection sites for at least 5 minutes.

Platelet transfusions are indicated prophylactically (purely on the basis of the platelet count) when there is a significant risk of haemorrhage arising from a further decline in the platelet count due to marrow failure, and the platelet count is already low ($<20 \times 10^9$/litre). This particularly applies to patients with acute leukaemia, and others with rapidly falling counts and with infections. Other more stable patients may tolerate platelet counts $<10 \times 10^9$/litre very well and do not require routine prophylactic transfusion purely on the basis of the platelet count; prophylactic administration is required prior to surgery if the count is $<75 \times 10^9$/litre. Transfusions are indicated therapeutically for patients with counts $<20 \times 10^9$/litre in the presence of frank bleeding (but not necessarily as a routine in patients with mild purpura), or retinal haemorrhages (the retina is an extension of the CNS). The fundi and skin must be examined daily in these patients, and the urine checked for red blood cells.

Six pooled units of platelet concentrate are usually given at any one time, repeated daily, or more frequently, as necessary. Anti-platelet antibodies may develop with a consequent decline in the efficacy of repeated transfusions. Ideally transfused platelets should be at least ABO compatible; HLA-compatible platelets (collected from a single donor by cell separator) are preferable if frequent transfusion appears likely and if the efficacy of transfusions is declining.

The cytotoxic drug vincristine has minimal marrow toxicity and can actually raise the platelet count. This may be either as a result of binding to platelets with consequent selective toxicity at reticulo-endothelial sites of sequestration or destruction, or due to the inhibition of megakaryocyte mitosis acting as a stimulus to their endoreduplication.

## Thrombocytosis

Causes include polycythaemia rubra vera, chronic granulocytic leukaemia, chronic haemorrhage, infection, surgery and splenectomy. More commonly, however, it is found as a para-neoplastic phenomenon accompanying a wide range of cancers, usually those that are more advanced; it can also occur as a rebound phenomenon after cytotoxic chemotherapy. Counts above $1,000 \times 10^9$/litre carry a risk of both thrombosis and haemorrhage, but these occur very rarely. In addition to treatment directed against the underlying cause, cell separation may be considered for some patients, although the tendency to thrombosis can also be reduced with low-dose aspirin, 75 mg/day.

## Thrombosis

Causes include bed rest, surgery, dehydration, diuretics, stilboestrol, venous compression by tumour (particularly pelvic tumours), hyperviscosity, polycythaemia, thrombocytosis and a para-neoplastic, hypercoagulable state that can occur with pancreatic, lung and other cancers. Local thrombophlebitis is common following injection of cytotoxic drugs. Standard anticoagulant treatment is not usually successful in preventing paraneoplastic 'migratory thrombophlebitis'.

**NOTES**

# NOTES

# CHAPTER 12

# Immunosuppres-
# sion and
# Infections

Cancer, cytotoxic chemotherapy, radiotherapy and even surgery are all potentially immunosuppressive. Particularly immunosuppressive malignancies are those which are lymphoproliferative or myeloproliferative, including multiple myeloma and Hodgkin's disease. Although immunosuppression does occur with carcinomas it is usually much less profound. In general the more aggressive the neoplasm or its treatment with cytotoxic chemotherapy or very extensive radiotherapy the more profound will be the immunosuppression. Immunosuppression may involve quantitative and qualitative deficiencies in neutrophils, T- and B-lymphocytes, macrophages and natural killer cells.

Significant immunosuppression in cancer patients not only renders the host susceptible to infection with both common and otherwise rare organisms including bacteria, viruses and fungi but in addition the course of the infection can be extremely rapid, leading very quickly to a marked decline and death; approximately 10 per cent of infections in neutropenic patients are fatal. Many of these patients are, in addition, particularly susceptible to micro-organisms gaining entry to their body by virtue of the breakdown of skin and mucous membrane barriers by cytotoxic drug or radiation-induced mucositis – particularly affecting the alimentary tract; catheters, other invasive interventions and tumour infiltration are also sites of entry. Most viral infections in these patients are due to re-activation of latent herpes and hepatitis viruses.

Competent management of these patients involves a meticulous approach to sterile procedures, sometimes barrier nursing, alertness to the possibility of infection and informing patients of the vital necessity of very prompt reporting of any fever or other potentially suspicious symptoms. Often empirical broad-spectrum treatment must be instigated before a specific microbiological diagnosis has been made.

A specific microbiological diagnosis is quite often difficult. Bacteria are not always isolated and because of the immunosuppression the rôle of serology is limited: negative titres do not necessarily exclude a specific infection. Biopsy specimens and the use of special stains, immunofluorescence or electron microscopy are quite often required for the diagnosis of non-bacterial infections.

# Prevention of Infection

## Hygiene

Patients at high risk of infection, particularly those who are receiving intensive cytotoxic chemotherapy and who are severely leucopenic, should ideally be nursed in isolation, although the benefit from this by itself is limited. Staff and other visitors entering the room should wear gowns and masks and adopt a meticulous approach to hand-washing. All food should be thoroughly cooked, as uncooked foods can be a source of several potential pathogens. Soft ripened cheeses (not processed or cottage cheeses or spreads) should be avoided as they can be a source of *Listeria monocytogenes*. Patients should also be advised strongly to reheat cook-chilled meals purchased at retail outlets, and ready-to-eat poultry, to reduce the risk of contamination by this organism which can cause septicaemia and meningitis in the immunocompromised.

'Total protection' with the use of purpose-built laminar air flow rooms with high-efficiency air filters provides some additional protection, particularly from infection with aspergillus; such units are however very expensive both to build and to run. Immunosuppressed patients not receiving intensive treatment are usually much safer at home than in hospital, where they may be more likely to contract some infections, including some that may be relatively resistant to treatment.

Attention to the sterility of procedures is very important, including thorough hand-washing and the wearing of gloves. Attention should also regularly be given to the care and changing of intravenous cannulae and urinary catheters, and to oral hygiene.

## Screening of blood products

Screening for HBsAg is now routine and the risk of transmission of hepatitis B is extremely low. Cytomegalovirus infections are quite common in patients receiving unscreened fresh blood or granulocyte concentrates (the virus dies after a few days' storage) and they can be fulminating in immunosuppressed patients, particularly bone marrow transplant recipients.

## Chemoprophylaxis

Prophylactic drug treatment can lessen the risk of some infections in patients undergoing severely marrow-suppressive therapy. The rôle of prophylactic antibiotics remains very controversial. There is declining enthusiasm for attempting gut decontamination with oral non-absorbable regimens such as FRACON (framycetin, colistin and nystatin). Various regimens of systemic antibiotics have been used, but there is concern about the induction of resistant strains and about problems arising from marrow suppression by regimens containing co-trimoxazole. Co-trimoxazole is of particular value in the prevention of *Pneumocystis carinii* pneumonia, but the inhalation of a pentamidine aerosol once per month has also been shown to reduce the incidence of *Pneumocystis carinii* pneumonia, without significant side effects. If prophylactic antibiotics are given they should be started just before the neutropenia with the initiation of intensive treatment, and continued until the granulocyte count rises to $1 \times 10^9$/litre.

Oral amphotericin B or nystatin lozenges, or ketoconazole or miconazole gel, in conjunction with excellent oral hygiene, may help to prevent mucosal candidiasis and secondary bacterial infection. This may also lessen the risk of systemic candidiasis. Anti-viral prophylaxis is now feasible and appropriate for high-risk groups, particularly patients receiving bone marrow transplantation and induction chemotherapy for leukaemia. Acyclovir given intravenously (10 mg/kg tds) or orally (400–800 mg qds) has been shown to reduce substantially the incidence of herpes simplex infection; it also gives protection against varicella zoster.

## Immunoprophylaxis

Active immunisation has little value in these patients because they are immunosuppressed, and all live vaccines should be avoided at all costs on a long-term basis. Polyvalent pneumococcal vaccine can however reduce the chance of subsequent pneumococcal infection in patients who have had a splenectomy. Pneumococcal septicaemia can be rapidly fatal in splenectomised patients: without prophylaxis 2–3 per cent will die from it. The vaccine should be given ≥2 weeks before the spleen is removed. It covers approximately 90 per cent of the pneumococci that cause serious infection. Revaccination should be avoided as it can cause a serious reaction. Passive immunisation with zoster immune globulin given to patients without herpes zoster antibodies within 72 hours of contact affords some short-lived protection (6 weeks), however it is not easily available.

### Avoidance of live vaccines

These can cause very severe infections in patients who are immunosuppressed through receiving cytotoxic chemotherapy or wide-field radiotherapy for any malignancy, and should be avoided during treatment and for probably at least a year afterwards. Patients who have been treated for leukaemia, Hodgkin's disease and non-Hodgkin's lymphoma can be immunosuppressed many years after successful treatment and the administration of live vaccines can be hazardous at any time after treatment.

*Vaccines containing live organisms:* BCG; mumps; live poliomyelitis; rubella; yellow fever.

*Vaccines not containing live organisms:* cholera; diphtheria; hepatitis B; influenza; pertussis; pneumococcus; inactivated poliomyelitis; tetanus; typhoid.

### Cytokines

Granulocyte and granulocyte-monocyte colony stimulating factors (G-CSF:GM-CSF) may have a rôle in the lessening of cytopenic infection, but this is not yet fully defined. They can shorten the pancytopenic period following bone marrow transplantation, but should not be used in patients with AML or CGL because of the possibility of stimulation of the leukaemic cells.

# Management of Suspected Infection (Especially with Neutropenia)

Fever is the most common initial manifestation of infection in immunosuppressed patients and is almost always due to infection and not the underlying malignancy. It is important to remember that fever is not inevitable in severe infection, particularly in patients on high dose steroids, and infection should always be considered in any unexplained deterioration (e.g. hypotension). In addition, even in the presence of fever, localising symptoms and signs may be absent or minimal because of the impaired immune response, e.g. classical abscess formation may not take place due to the lack of white blood cells, and peritonitis may cause only mild abdominal tenderness.

In this context infection very commonly occurs in patients who are neutropenic. The risk of infection rises rapidly with neutrophil counts $<1.0 \times 10^9$/litre. Patients with suspected infection should be questioned and examined very carefully indeed, with particular attention to skin, entry sites of intravenous catheters, mouth and oropharynx, gut, anus (rectal examination should not normally be performed because of the risk of stimulating entry of organisms into the blood stream), chest, urinary tract, meninges and heart valves.

## Investigations

Blood should be taken promptly for aerobic and anaerobic bacterial culture, and fungal culture. A sample should also be saved as a baseline for serology, although this is often of limited value because of the immunosuppression. In patients with an indwelling venous catheter samples for blood culture should be taken through the catheter as well as from a peripheral vein. An MSU and throat swab should be taken together with swabs from any sites that are obviously, or possibly, infected; these should be sent for bacterial and viral culture. In addition to cultures, direct microscopy of sputum, pus or any other suspicious secretion with bacterial (Gram) and fungal staining may quickly provide very useful information. Another important investigation is a chest X-ray.

## Anti-microbial treatment

Intravenous broad-spectrum antibiotic therapy should be instituted in neutropenic patients if the temperature rises above 38°C for 2 hours and in some patients after a single high reading, particularly if it is >38.5°C or there are other signs of deterioration, without waiting for a specific microbiological diagnosis. Although the mortality risk from infection in these patients is approximately 10 per cent overall, it is substantially higher in the presence of shock, raised blood urea and poor general condition.

A variety of drugs and combinations may be appropriate and it is sometimes best to obtain local microbiological advice. Gram-negative bacteraemia, especially with *Pseudomonas*, carries a very substantial risk of morbidity and mortality. Other common bacterial infections include *E. coli*, *Klebsiella*, *Staphylococcus aureus* and *Streptococci*, and mixed infections may occur in these patients. Anaerobic bacterial infections are somewhat less common. The possibility of reactivation of tuberculosis should never be forgotten.

A combination of an anti-pseudomonal penicillin (e.g. piperacillin, azlocillin) with an aminoglycoside (e.g. gentamicin, netilmicin, tobramicin, amikacin) will usually give very satisfactory cover against these organisms. Alternatively third-generation cephalosporins (e.g. ceftazidime) may be used instead of a broad-spectrum penicillin. Another newer broad-spectrum antibiotic is the quinolone ciprofloxacin, however there has been some concern about the induction of multiple resistance with some of the newer antibiotics. Attention to renal excretion is important and serum peak and trough aminoglycoside levels must be measured to ensure the achievement of concentrations in the therapeutic range and avoid a high risk of nephrotoxicity and ototoxicity. Prolonged treatment with aminoglycosides can also cause hypomagnesaemic tetany. Ceftazidime levels should also be monitored in patients with renal impairment. Treatment should be continued for 3 days after the disappearance of pyrexia.

Failure to see a satisfactory response to initial broad-spectrum antibiotic therapy by 48 hours should prompt reassessment. By then an organism may have been isolated and sensitivity established; alternative therapy may therefore be indicated. A change in regimen should be considered if no organism has been isolated, after taking further specimens for microbiology. A vancomycin-containing regimen should be particularly considered in patients at risk of Gram-positive infection from an indwelling venous line or quinolone prophylaxis. Cephalosporins have activity against anaerobic bacteria but metronidazole is the drug of choice. If there has been no satisfactory clinical response by 4–5 days and still no organism has been isolated, serious consideration should be given to starting empirical antifungal therapy with amphotericin B. The symptoms and signs of invasive fungal infection (usually candidiasis or aspergillosis) are non-specific, and less than 10 per cent of these infections are currently identified before death (see section on non-bacterial infections below).

## Other measures

Infection of the tunnel of a Hickman line is usually considered an indication for its removal, but this is not necessary if only the entry site is infected.

Granulocyte transfusions are not easily available, but may be considered in the face of continuing severe leucopenia and infection (see section on haematological disturbances). The rôle of these transfusions remains controversial, but if possible an ABO matched motivated family donor should be used.

## Management of shock

Bacteraemia, particularly with Gram-negative organisms, can cause shock with a consequent high risk of death. A successful outcome may depend not only on antibiotic therapy, but also on meticulous monitoring and supportive care. Monitoring will include assessments of renal function, blood-gas and acid-base status, cardiovascular status (including central venous or pulmonary artery pressure), full blood count, prothrombin ratio and KCCT. Treatment includes the maintenance of an adequate cardiac output with fluid infusion and possibly dopamine or noradrenaline, oxygen (and if necessary ventilation), and replacement of clotting factors (fresh plasma or fresh frozen plasma is a useful fluid). The use of high dose steroids remains controversial unless there is adrenal insufficiency, which may be suggested by a raised or even normal lymphocyte count.

# Non-bacterial Infections

## Herpes simplex

Labial and oro-pharyngeal ulceration are the most common manifestations. Herpes simplex quite commonly causes stomatitis in the absence of classical vesicles. Other manifestations include ano-genital infection, oesophagitis, ophthalmitis, encephalitis, hepatitis and pneumonitis. The diagnosis is best confirmed by electron microscopy or immunofluorescence of vesicle fluid, scrapings or biopsy material. Prompt administration of acyclovir 5–10 mg/kg 8 hourly IV for 7 days reduces the duration of virus shedding, accelerates healing and prevents dissemination. Five per cent acyclovir cream may be sufficient for herpes labialis in less severely immunosuppressed patients.

## Herpes zoster

Shingles is quite common in cancer patients and the characteristic rash is usually preceded by pain in the affected dermatome(s) for several days. In severely immunosuppressed patients shingles carries a high risk of dissemination but the rash is often disseminated from the outset. Pneumonitis and encephalitis are other manifestations. Prompt administration of acyclovir 10 mg/kg 8 hourly IV for 7 days reduces the duration of virus shedding and halts progression.

## Cytomegalovirus

This infection can be transmitted by blood transfusion. The diagnosis is usually established by the identification of characteristic intranuclear inclusions on biopsy material. Clinical features include oesophagitis, pneumonitis, colitis, and haemolytic anaemia. There is now good evidence of efficacy for an acyclovir analogue, ganciclovir. This is given by intravenous infusion, 5 mg/kg over 1 hour every 12 hours for 14–21 days, with dose reduction in the presence of renal insufficiency. Marrow suppression is common and the full blood count must be closely monitored. There may be additive toxicity with the concurrent administration of cytotoxic drugs and amphotericin B or co-trimoxazole.

## Fungi

Oropharyngeal candidiasis usually responds well to very frequent (2-hourly during the waking hours) topical treatment with amphotericin B or nystatin lozenges. Miconazole gel or ketoconazole oral suspension has a systemic effect as well as a local one, but nevertheless should be kept in the mouth for as long as possible. A convenient alternative systemic treatment is fluconazole capsules given only once daily for 7–14 days.

Invasive fungal infections are often first suspected when fever does not respond to broad-spectrum antibacterial therapy. The commonest infections are *Candida albicans* and *Aspergillus fumigatus*. There are now sensitive methods available for the detection of circulating candida antigens using enzyme-linked immunosorbent assay (ELISA), radio-immuno-assay and a technically easier agglutination test. Candidiasis can involve almost any organ but those more commonly involved include the lungs, oesophagus, kidneys and liver. The main site of infection in aspergillosis is the lungs, sometimes with infarction. The yeast *Cryptococcus neoformans* causes meningitis, often with an insidious onset of headache and mental changes.

The drug of choice for these infections remains amphotericin B, 0.25 mg/kg daily increasing to a maximum of 1.5 mg/kg daily by intravenous infusion; it can also be given intrathecally. It is an unpleasant drug causing nausea, vomiting, local thrombophlebitis, fever, hypokalaemia and nephrotoxicity. Urinary function should be monitored closely and the dosage must be reduced if there is an increasing serum urea or creatinine concentration. The addition of a small amount of heparin to the infusion may help to lessen thrombophlebitis. The concomitant administration of other potentially nephrotoxic drugs should be avoided. Treatment should be continued for a minimum of two weeks.

Flucytosine 150 mg/kg/day in 4 divided doses, intravenously or orally, may be given in addition to amphotericin, with which there is some synergy. Its good penetration into urine and CSF is of potential benefit. The dose should be reduced in renal failure and marrow depression can occur. Resistance to this drug is quite common, particularly in the USA, and if possible sensitivity testing should be performed.

The imidazole drugs (miconazole 600 mg 8 hourly by intravenous infusion or ketoconazole 200–400 mg once daily by mouth) have activity against systemic fungal infections but their rôle has not been clearly established: they may have a rôle in prophylaxis. They may be considered as second-line drugs but have no activity against aspergillus. A new agent, itraconazole, does possess useful activity against aspergillus, which is not always responsive to amphotericin.

## Pneumocystis carinii

This organism is now also considered to be a fungus. In most cases infection probably results from reactivation of latent organisms. Common features are a dry cough, swinging pyrexia and marked dyspnoea and tachypnoea, usually with minimal signs on lung auscultation. The chest X-ray commonly shows diffuse bilateral parenchymal infiltration, but cavitation can occur. Cyanosis and respiratory failure can supervene quite rapidly.

*Some common antibiotics*

| Drug | Adult dosage in immunosuppression | Comments |
|------|-----------------------------------|----------|
| Amikacin | 15 mg/kg/day given 12-hourly IV injection over 2 minutes or IM | Side effects include nephrotoxicity and ototoxicity. Dosage should be reduced in renal impairment: the required interval in hours between doses may be estimated by multiplying the serum creatinine concentration in *mg/100 ml* by 9 or by dividing the concentration in *micromol/l* by 10. Plasma concentrations should be monitored. |
| Azlocillin | 3 g every 4 hours IV injection over 3 minutes or infusion over 30 minutes | Dose should be reduced in renal impairment; given every 12 hours if creatinine clearance <30 ml/min (serum creatinine >200 micromol/l). |
| Carbenicillin | 5 g every 4 hours IV injection over 3 minutes or infusion over 30 minutes | Rich in sodium. Can cause hypokalaemia. Dose should be reduced in renal impairment; 3 g every 4 hours if creatinine clearance 10–50 ml/min (serum creatinine 150–400 micromol/l) and further if necessary. |
| Cefotaxime | 2.0 g every 8 hours IV or IM injection or infusion over 30 minutes | Dosage should only be reduced in severe renal failure; by 50 per cent if serum creatinine >750 micromol/l. |

| | | |
|---|---|---|
| Ceftazidime | 2 g every 8 hours IV or IM injection | Dosage should be reduced in renal impairment: 1.5 g every 12 hours if creatinine clearance 30–50 ml/min (serum creatinine 150–200 micromol/l); every 24 hours if 15–30 ml/min (serum creatinine 200–350 micromol/l) and further if necessary. Serum levels should be monitored in patients with renal impairment and pre-dose concentration should not exceed 40 mg/litre. |
| Ciproflaxacin | 200 mg 12 hourly IV infusion over 30 minutes | Dosage should be reduced in renal impairment but only if creatinine clearance falls below 20 ml/minute. |
| Co-trimoxazole | 960 mg bd (conventional and prophylactic oral dose) 120 mg/kg/day therapeutic for pneumocystis by IV infusion over 90 minutes: ampoules must be diluted just before use | Side effects include marrow suppression and folate deficiency. Dosage should be reduced in renal impairment: halve conventional dosage if creatinine clearance 15–25 ml/min (serum creatinine 200–400 micromol/l) and further if necessary. As therapy for pneumocystis serum concentration should be ≥5 micrograms/ml. |
| Gentamicin | 5 mg/kg/day given 8-hourly IV injection over 2 minutes or IM | Side effects include nephrotoxicity and ototoxicity. Dose must be reduced in renal impairment: 12-hourly interval between doses if creatinine clearance 30–70 ml/min (blood urea 6–17 mmol/l); 24 hours for 10–30 ml/min (blood urea 17–34 mmol/l) and further if necessary. Plasma concentrations must be monitored. One hour after injection; this |

*Some common antibiotics*

| Drug | Adult dosage in immunosuppression | Comments |
|------|-----------------------------------|----------|
| | | should not exceed 10 micrograms/ml and pre-dose level should be under 2 micrograms/ml |
| Metronidazole | 500 mg 8-hourly<br>IV infusion over 20 minutes | No dose reduction for renal failure. |
| Netilmicin | 7.5 mg/kg/day 8-hourly<br>Reduce to 6 mg after 48 hours<br>IV injection over 3 minutes or infusion over 30–120 minutes or IM | Side effects include nephrotoxicity and ototoxicity. Dose should be reduced in renal impairment. Initial dosage should be reduced by 20 per cent if serum creatinine 100–120 micromol/l, by 50 per cent if creatinine 180–190 micromol/l, by 80 per cent if creatinine 365–450 micromol/l and further if necessary. Plasma concentrations should be monitored. |
| Piperacillin | 3 g every 4 hours<br>IV injection over 3 minutes or infusion over 30 minutes | Dose should be reduced in marked renal impairment: 1 g every 4 hours if creatinine clearance <10 ml/min (serum creatinine >400 micromol/l). |

| | | |
|---|---|---|
| Ticarcillin | 3 g every 4 hours<br>IV injection over 3 minutes or infusion over 30 minutes | Should not be mixed in same bottle with aminoglycosides. Dosage should be reduced in renal impairment: 2.0 g every 4 hours if creatinine clearance 10–50 ml/min (serum creatinine 150–400 micromol/l) and further if necessary. |
| Tobramycin | 5 mg/kg/day given 8-hourly<br>IV or IM injection | As for gentamicin. |
| Vancomycin | 500 mg every 6 hours<br>IV infusion over 20–30 minutes | Side effects include nephrotoxicity and ototoxicity. Dosage should be reduced in renal impairment: 1.0 g every 36 hours if creatinine clearance 10–50 ml/min (serum creatinine 150–400 micromol/l) and further if necessary. |

The organisms are only rarely identified by conventional staining of routinely obtained sputum specimens, and the preferred method for establishing the diagnosis has been by bronchial brushing, bronchoalveolar lavage and/or transbronchial biopsy at bronchoscopy. Immunofluorescent staining with a monoclonal antibody appears to be considerably more sensitive than the other methods of demonstrating infection in some ordinary sputum specimens. Deep sputum specimens for this technique can be achieved non-invasively in some patients following the inhalation of hypertonic saline. Treatment is often instigated empirically however on the basis of the clinical and radiological features.

The drug of choice is co-trimoxazole in high dosage – 120 mg/kg daily by intravenous injection in 4 divided doses for 14 days. This is usually well tolerated but can cause marrow suppression. Some non-responding patients will respond to pentamidine. When given systemically this is very toxic – there is now evidence that it is effective and much better tolerated (except for irritation and coughing) if given in a nebulised form.

**NOTES**

**NOTES**

# CHAPTER 13

# Metabolic Disturbances

## Ectopic ACTH Syndrome

See also section on hypokalaemia. In patients with small cell carcinomas the ectopic ACTH syndrome usually signifies an appalling prognosis: plasma ACTH and cortisol levels are usually very high, the plasma potassium concentration is usually well below 3 mmol/litre, and there is also frank diabetes mellitus. Oedema and pigmentation are very common but these patients rarely live long enough to develop the classical clinical features of Cushing's syndrome.

Management of these patients depends on the clinical situation. Enthusiastic attempts to suppress plasma cortisol levels and control diabetes may not be justified in patients with widespread metastases. However, in patients with a more readily treatable bronchial carcinoid tumour or apparently localised small cell carcinoma, attention to endocrine status will be justified until the anticipated benefit from surgery, chemotherapy or radiotherapy is achieved.

Metyrapone inhibits 11β-hydroxylation in the adrenal cortex and is sometimes of benefit in reducing cortisol production, but rarely in ectopic ACTH secretion from small cell carcinomas. A reasonable dose is 1–1.5 g qds. Adrenal cortisol excretion may also be reduced by aminoglutethimide (250 mg qds), which inhibits the conversion of cholesterol to pregnenolone. This drug quite often causes drowsiness and a rash, but both usually subside with continued administration. Rare patients with indolent incurable tumours may benefit from bilateral adrenalectomy.

# Hypercalcaemia

This is a common electrolytic disturbance in cancer patients. It is most frequently due to multiple bone metastases but occasionally it is due to secretion of parathormone-like or other humoral agents by a tumour which has not spread to bone, most commonly a squamous carcinoma of bronchus. The pathogenesis of hypercalcaemia involves increased bone resorption and/or increased renal tubular calcium reabsorption. There is a tendency for the former to be the principal factor in hypercalcaemia from metastatic osteolysis from breast carcinoma and myeloma, and the latter in non-metastatic hypercalcaemia due to squamous carcinoma of the bronchus and renal carcinoma, and in breast cancer patients with liver metastases. Intestinal absorption of calcium is rarely significant in pathogenesis and a low-calcium diet is of little therapeutic benefit.

In patients with an underlying tendency to hypercalcaemia it may be precipitated by dehydration (e.g. from reduced fluid intake; vomiting; diarrhoea), and by immobilisation (e.g. from hospitalisation; pathological fracture) which increases bone resorption. Endocrine manipulations in patients with metastatic breast carcinoma, particularly the introduction of tamoxifen, can also occasionally precipitate hypercalcaemia. This may be part of a 'flare' phenomenon and it may presage a subsequent useful tumour response.

The common clinical features of hypercalcaemia are nausea, vomiting, malaise, constipation, confusion, weakness, polyuria, thirst and dehydration: it causes a nephrogenic diabetes insipidus. Symptoms can often be present with only minor elevations of serum calcium and the pain threshold may be lowered.

The management should depend on the clinical situation. Enthusiastic treatment may be inappropriate, especially for patients who cannot be expected to benefit from any treatment directed against their cancer and who are terminally ill. Nevertheless the presence of distressing symptoms may justify attempts to lower the serum calcium concentration and, where appropriate, treatment directed against the cancer (surgery or radiotherapy for non-metastatic hypercalcaemia, endocrine manipulation or cytotoxic drugs for patients with bone metastases) is likely to be crucial in achieving medium- or long-term normocalcaemia.

## Rehydration

This is the mainstay of initial treatment, usually achieved with intravenous fluids, unless the hypercalcaemia is mild. Normal saline, 1 litre 4 hourly with 20 mEq potassium chloride in each alternate litre is a reasonable initial replacement, but the urea and other electrolyte concentrations should be checked daily at the start of treatment, as well as the serum calcium. Frusemide 40–80 mg daily (but *not* a thiazide diuretic) blocks renal tubular calcium reabsorption, and may help to prevent fluid overload.

## Mobilisation

This should be enthusiastically pursued, since it reduces osteoclastic activity and increases osteoblastic activity. Where there is uncontrolled pain, the achievement of adequate analgesia is important to mobility.

## Drugs

### Diphosphonates

These drugs are analogues of pyrophosphate, a natural regulator of bone mineral precipitation and dissolution. They inhibit osteoclastic activity and, to a variable extent depending on the particular analogue, osteoblastic activity also. Whilst rehydration will increase renal calcium excretion, in the absence of other measures any excessive release of calcium from bone will continue unaffected. This release can be blocked with diphosphonates, but they take 3–4 days to achieve a near maximal response.

Diphosphonates are relatively free from serious toxicity. The duration of benefit from a single 3-day course of intravenous treatment is usually 1–2 weeks. Intravenous administrations may be repeated once, and further treatment is justified for some patients. Diphosphonates can improve metastatic bone pain in some patients, and there is also evidence that APD can cause recalcification of lytic metastases. Examples of diphosphonate regimens are:

Etidronate 7.5 mg/kg/day in 500 ml intravenous normal saline over 2 hours or more for 3 consecutive days, possibly followed by maintenance with 20 mg/kg/day orally for up to 3 months. Etidronate can cause transient taste loss.

Pamidronate (APD) intravenously in normal saline over 24 hours, total dose varying from 30 mg (serum calcium <3 mmol/l) to 90 mg (serum calcium >4 mmol/l).

Clodronate 500–1000 mg intravenously in normal saline over 8 hours.

## Calcitonin

Although this also works by inhibiting both osteoclastic activity and renal tubular calcium reabsorption, it is considerably more rapid in action than diphosphonates. An effect is usually seen within hours, but it is usually relatively short-lived, often lasting only 2–3 days; this may be due to down-regulation of receptors. Prolonged treatment is therefore not usually appropriate, although the addition of corticosteroids can help to delay refractoriness. As with the diphosphonates there can be a beneficial effect on metastatic bone pain in some patients. An acceptable regimen is salmon calcitonin 25–100 IU 6 hourly subcutaneously or intramuscularly for 2–3 days.

## Corticosteroids

These are usually of little value except in patients with lymphoproliferative malignancies (particularly multiple myeloma), and in some patients with breast carcinoma. Possible mechanisms include direct anti-tumour action, and suppression of prostaglandin synthesis, osteoclast activation or vitamin D metabolism. An acceptable regimen is enteric coated prednisolone 30–40 mg orally daily in divided doses.

## Mithramycin

This cytotoxic antibiotic inhibits bone resorption at a dose level below that required for an anti-tumour effect. It may also inhibit renal tubular calcium reabsorption. A single dose produces a maximal effect in 2–3 days, but this lasts only about one week. Prolonged administration carries a risk of bone marrow, renal and hepatic toxicity. A common regimen is 25 µg/kg body weight/day in 1 litre of 5 per cent dextrose infused intravenously over 4 hours for 3 consecutive days, but quite often a single dose will suffice.

### Phosphate

Oral phosphate is often helpful in maintaining normocalcaemia. It too may act by inhibiting or reversing bone resorption. Binding to dietary calcium within the gut is not likely to be an important mode of action since intestinal calcium absorption is rarely a significant factor in the pathogenesis of malignant hypercalcaemia. The maximum daily dose is 3 g (elemental phosphorus) and for longer-term treatment a reasonable daily dose is 1.5 g (elemental phosphorus). Large doses often cause diarrhoea and there is also a potential hazard of nephrocalcinosis. Apart from the risk of diarrhoea it is symptomatically very well tolerated, although in patients with renal impairment there should be a dose reduction.

### Prostaglandin synthetase inhibitors

These are probably helpful in correcting hypercalcaemia in some patients, perhaps especially those with squamous carcinomas without widespread bone metastases.

# Hyperglycaemia

In patients with latent diabetes this can be precipitated by reduced activity, and commonly by steroids. It is a feature of Cushing's syndrome and is often very marked in ectopic ACTH secretion (see separate section). Occasionally hyperglycaemia can occur as a result of pancreatitis due to asparaginase, and also following treatment with the cytotoxic drug streptozotocin which has some specificity for pancreatic endocrine cells.

# Hyperkalaemia

The commonest cause of severe hyperkalaemia in cancer patients is renal failure from obstruction caused by advanced intrapelvic tumour. Active treatment for such patients is not always justified (see section on renal failure). Hyperkalaemia is very occasionally caused by very rapid destruction of bulky tumour with chemotherapy for leukaemia or lymphoma (tumour lysis syndrome). Sometimes the reported hyperkalaemia can be spurious, due to the release of potassium from large numbers of leukaemic cells during *in vitro* clotting.

Emergency treatment may require the infusion of 10 units of soluble insulin in 100 ml of 50 per cent dextrose, which together promote the transfer of potassium into cells. The effect of hyperkalaemia on the heart can be counteracted by the intravenous injection of 20 ml 10 per cent calcium gluconate over 5–10 minutes. Another remedy, less rapid but suitable for medium-term control, is the oral or rectal administration of polystyrene sulphonate ion-exchange resins, e.g. calcium or sodium resonium 15 g tds orally or 30 g rectally daily. Calcium resin should be avoided in patients at risk for hypercalcaemia, and the sodium resin avoided in those with evidence of fluid overload or severe renal impairment. Peritoneal or haemodialysis for renal failure can rapidly correct hyperkalaemia.

# Hyperphosphataemia

Rapid tumour (leukaemia or lymphoma) lysis with cytotoxic chemotherapy can also precipitate hyperphosphataemia, although this may already be present as a result of rapid cell turnover. The hyperphosphataemia is not by itself symptomatic but it can cause hypocalcaemia and may be accompanied by hyperuricaemia.

# Hyperuricaemia

Rapid lysis of bulky tumour can release large amounts of nucleoproteins, resulting in excess production of uric acid. Hyperuricaemia can lead to precipitation of urate crystals within the renal tubules, causing acute renal failure. Fortunately this complication can usually be avoided by the prophylactic administration of allopurinol (100 mg tds), which should be started at least 12 hours prior to treatment. Good hydration is also important, and the urinary pH should be kept alkaline since this increases urate solubility. Allopurinol should be given whenever there is a possibility of rapid lysis of bulky neoplasms, usually with cytotoxic chemotherapy for acute leukaemia or lymphoma. Allopurinol can potentiate the effects of 6-mercaptopurine and azathioprine and their dosage should be reduced accordingly.

Patients with established urate nephropathy and oliguria (rather than anuria) should be treated with allopurinol and urinary alkalinisation, e.g. with intravenous 1.4 per cent sodium bicarbonate 500 ml 2–4 hourly or with oral sodium bicarbonate in water 5–10 g 2–4 hourly, in conjunction with frequent urinary pH monitoring and attention to fluid balance. Peritoneal or haemodialysis may be necessary, although the latter is more effective in removing uric acid from the blood.

# Hypocalcaemia

Mild hypocalcaemia is as at least as common in cancer patients with bone spread as is hypercalcaemia, occurring in patients with osteoblastic metastases, especially from prostate and breast carcinomas: it is very rarely symptomatic. Symptomatic hypocalcaemia (tetany) may occur after parathyroid damage (often temporary) or removal by thyroid surgery, and occasionally as a result of cisplatinum-induced hypomagnesaemia and from hyperphosphataemia in the tumour lysis syndrome (see separate sections). Hypocalcaemia may occur with osteomalacia as a rare complication of gastrectomy.

Tetany is treated with intravenous 10 per cent calcium gluconate (10 ml), followed if necessary by infusion of 40 ml daily; the serum calcium concentration should be closely monitored. Intravenous calcium must be given slowly – not more than 2 ml/min. Particular caution should be exercised in patients on digoxin. An early warning of too-rapid injection is oral tingling and a general feeling of warmth.

Hypoparathyroidism may be treated initially with oral calcium gluconate tablets 5–20 g daily and calciferol 50,000–200,000 units daily. Continued calcium supplementation is rarely required for persisting parathyroidism.

# Hypoglycaemia

This should be thought of in any patient with confusion, drowsiness or loss of consciousness. Occasionally this may be precipitated by poor nutritional intake secondary to anorexia, nausea or vomiting. It can also occur as a complication of gastrectomy. It is the characteristic feature of pancreatic insulinoma and may also occur (although very rarely) as a paraneoplastic phenomenon with other tumours, e.g. bulky soft tissue sarcomas, Hodgkin's disease, acute leukaemia, carcinoid tumours and in patients with very extensive liver involvement. Mechanisms may include elaboration of insulin-like humoral agents by the tumour, autoantibodies to insulin receptors, uptake of glucose by bulky tumour and interference with hepatic gluconeogenesis. Streptozotocin (see hyperglycaemia) can occasionally cause transient initial hypoglycaemia due to sudden insulin release from damaged pancreatic islet cells.

# Hypokalaemia

Common causes are diuretics, steroids, laxatives, diarrhoea and vomiting. Less common causes include alkalosis and nephropathies. A rare but more specifically oncological cause is the excessive endogenous mineralocorticoid excretion which occurs in Conn's and Cushing's syndromes and in ectopic ACTH syndrome (see separate section). The rare paraneoplastic causes of diarrhoea include medullary carcinoma of thyroid, carcinoid syndrome and tumours secreting vasoactive intestinal polypeptide ('vipomas') producing the 'WDHA' syndrome – watery diarrhoea, hypokalaemia and achlorhydria.

Hypokalaemia may cause weakness, ileus and digoxin toxicity. For most patients oral supplementation with 10–15 g potassium chloride daily (135–200 mmol) is sufficient, but severe hypokalaemia requires intravenous correction. Potassium chloride solutions should not contain more than 40 mmol/litre and they should be given slowly (not more than 1 litre 4-hourly). Intravenous dosages of more than 80 mmol/day should only be given if indicated by repeated plasma electrolyte measurement.

# Hypomagnesaemia

Cisplatin can cause renal magnesium loss. Hypomagnesaemia (sometimes prolonged) is very common in patients receiving this drug, particularly in those who also suffer severe vomiting which can contribute to magnesium deficiency. The normal range of serum magnesium is 1.5–2.5 mmol/l, but levels down to 0.5 mmol/l are usually asymptomatic. Symptoms include tetany, cramp, weakness, paraesthesiae, cold extremities and dizziness; very occasionally fits, psychosis and coma may occur. Hypomagnesaemia impairs parathyroid function and there is usually associated hypocalcaemia. Hypokalaemia can also occur.

Magnesium may be given intravenously if necessary e.g. 50 mmol magnesium chloride or sulphate in 1 litre normal saline or 5 per cent glucose over 12–24 hours, and intravenous prophylaxis should be attempted in patients for whom hypomagnesaemia has been a problem, e.g. 10–20 mmol in 1 litre normal saline given as pre-treatment hydration. Magnesium may conveniently be given orally in the form of magnesium glycerophosphate 3–6 g daily (12–24 mmol Mg), or magnesium citrate syrup, with little diarrhoea. Magnesium hydroxide is less well absorbed and causes more diarrhoea.

It has been reported that routine intravenous magnesium supplementation with each administration of cisplatin, together with regular oral administration in-between pulses, can not only prevent symptomatic hypomagnesaemia but may reduce drug-induced renal damage.

# Hyponatraemia

Clinically important hyponatraemia in cancer patients is most commonly due to the 'syndrome' of inappropriate secretion of antidiuretic hormone (SIADH) (see separate section). Other causes of hyponatraemia include diuretics and adrenal or pituitary insufficiency, both of which may be caused by neoplasia.

# Hypophosphataemia

Hypophosphataemia (±osteomalacia) has been described as a paraneoplastic phenomenon in a variety of tumours, perhaps due to decreased endogenous synthesis of 1,25-dihydroxy-cholecalciferol. Hypophosphataemia is quite a common finding in patients with advanced carcinoma of the prostate, and appears to be responsible for muscle weakness and pain attributable to osteomalacia in addition to metastatic bone disease. Correction of the hypophosphataemia with 1–2 micrograms alfacalcidol or calcitriol daily can result in improvement of both pain and weakness.

# Lactic Acidosis

This can occur in any patient who is in severe shock or hypoxia and is almost always a terminal event. It is also a rare complication of malignancy *per se*, particularly leukaemia and lymphoma with extensive liver involvement. In this case the clinical manifestations are variable and non-specific, but may include hyperventilation, malaise, weakness, nausea, vomiting and drowsiness. The clue to diagnosis is a high anion gap [$(Na^+ + K^+)$ minus $(Cl^- + HCO_3^-)$]. The normal anion gap is 10–18 mmol/l. The diagnosis is confirmed by the finding of a raised serum lactate (>2 mmol/l) which is probably due in most cases to the combination of production of lactate by glycolysis in tumour tissue and impaired removal by the liver.

Successful treatment of the underlying malignancy will usually result in correction of the acidosis. However, severe acidosis (blood pH <7.1) may be treated with 1.26 per cent–1.4 per cent sodium bicarbonate solution infused at an initial rate of 500 ml/hour up to a total volume of about 2 litres; close monitoring of the blood pH is important. The addition of normal saline may help as there is usually co-existent sodium depletion, and correction of this restores the ability of the kidneys to produce bicarbonate. Less severe acidosis may respond well to normal saline alone, e.g. 1 litre 4–6 hourly, but there should be careful attention to the possibility of fluid overload.

# Renal Failure

The commonest cause of renal failure in cancer patients is obstructive nephropathy due to extensive intrapelvic or retroperitoneal tumour. Other causes relevant to malignancy include hypercalcaemia, hyperuricaemia, septicaemia, renal light chain deposition in myeloma, infiltration by lymphoma, amyloid, drugs (e.g. cisplatin, high dose methotrexate, aminoglycosides), disseminated intravascular coagulation, inferior vena caval thrombosis and radiation nephritis.

The management of renal failure depends on the clinical situation. If the underlying malignancy is considered readily treatable enthusiastic management of acute renal failure is almost always justified and recovery of renal function can usually be expected. In patients with an otherwise poor prognosis it may be unkind to attempt to reverse the effects of renal failure; purely symptomatic care may be far more appropriate.

Urinary tract obstruction due to Hodgkin's disease, non-Hodgkin's lymphoma and metastatic testicular tumours will often respond rapidly to treatment with radiotherapy or cytotoxic chemotherapy, but it is essential to consider the impact of renal failure on drug excretion. Obstruction due to carcinoma (particularly advanced squamous carcinoma of cervix) is often relieved with radiotherapy but usually rather more slowly, over a period of several days or a week or two. Dexamethasone (e.g. 4 mg tds) is probably a reasonable addition in most patients, since reduction of even a slight component of oedema within the tumour may help relieve pressure on the urinary tract.

Whilst waiting for anti-neoplastic measures to work, amelioration of uraemia and hyperkalaemia is essential. In particular hyperkalaemia can often increase precipitously to potentially fatal levels. A low protein and potassium diet and ion-exchange resins can be helpful, but are usually insufficient. For many patients more robust approaches to lessen the metabolic upset are appropriate. These comprise peritoneal or haemodialysis and, in patients with post-renal failure, a percutaneous nephrostomy or cystoscopic insertion of ureteric stent(s). Such measures can facilitate the administration of chemotherapy.

# Syndrome of Inappropriate ADH Secretion (SIADH)

See also section on hyponatraemia. This syndrome should never be diagnosed until impaired adrenal function has been definitely excluded. The commonest neoplastic cause is small cell carcinoma of the bronchus, although it has been described with many other tumours. Other causes of SIADH comprise a variety of CNS disorders (including brain tumour), chest disorders (including pneumonia), drugs (including vinca alkaloids and cyclophosphamide) and hypothyroidism.

Symptoms and signs usually only occur when the plasma sodium concentration is under 120 mmol/litre, and only become severe when it falls below 110 mmol/litre. They include nausea, vomiting, weakness, irritability, confusion, fits and coma.

The diagnosis of SIADH depends on the presence of hyponatraemia in conjunction with a urine osmolality greater than that of the plasma, normal renal and adrenal function, persistent urinary sodium excretion despite the hyponatraemia, and lack of hypovolaemia, hypotension and oedemaforming pathology. Hyponatraemia can result from adrenal metastases, particularly in patients with lung cancer.

The management of SIADH depends on the clinical situation. Mild to moderate hyponatraemia requires no treatment. For patients with readily treatable causative conditions an enthusiastic attempt to correct more severe hyponatraemia is justified. It may not be justified in patients who are terminally ill from the underlying cause: purely symptomatic management may be kinder.

Fluid restriction to under 1 litre/day is often effective but can be very unpleasant. The tetracycline antibiotic demeclocycline induces a partial nephrogenic diabetes insipidus and can be very useful in the correction of hyponatraemia, whilst obviating the need for fluid restriction. The recommended dose is initially 900–1,200 mg daily in divided doses, and 600–900 mg daily if longer-term maintenance is required. Its maximal effect may be delayed for up to 3–6 weeks. This drug can cause photosensitivity.

In the emergency of life-threatening profound hyponatraemia the infusion of hypertonic saline with frusemide is justified, but the benefit from this is usually short lived since the infused sodium is rapidly excreted. However, there has been some success reported with a regimen of 40 mg frusemide daily together with sodium chloride supplementation of 3–6 g daily.

**NOTES**

# NOTES

# CHAPTER 14

# Other Common Cancer Complications

## Ascites

Common causes are ovarian, large bowel, breast, gastric and pancreatic carcinoma. Frequently there is extensive peritoneal and omental involvement by exudative tumour, although obstruction to drainage by metastatic blockage of diaphragmatic lymphatics is probably important in most patients; for some patients another component is hypoalbuminaemia. Non-neoplastic causes must be considered in patients with negative cytology.

Occasionally the ascites is milky in appearance and is termed 'chylous'. This is due to the presence of lymph as a result of disease obstructing and disrupting major lymphatic vessels. Occasionally this can result from surgical damage, particularly retroperitoneal lymphadenectomy.

### Paracentesis

This relieves distension, dyspnoea due to splinting of the diaphragms and any consequent bowel obstruction. It should be carried out very carefully as a sterile procedure since ascites is a good bacterial medium. The trocha should be inserted without undue pressure, and with the hands placed so as to prevent any possibility of a sudden deep penetration. Great care should be taken to avoid hepatomegaly (or splenomegaly). Visceromegaly may be impossible to palpate in the presence of very extensive ascites: in general the left flank is safer than the right. For patients with extensive ascites the fluid should be drained slowly over 24 hours, using tube clamping. Rapid drainage can occasionally precipitate a rapid and unexplained profound decline in cardiovascular status.

### Anti-cancer treatment

Systemic treatment may be considered appropriate for the underlying malignancy. Ovarian carcinomas often respond well to cytotoxic chemotherapy and breast carcinomas quite often respond to hormonal manipulation or cytotoxic chemotherapy. For most of the other common malignant causes systemic cytotoxic chemotherapy is of limited value. Some benefit has been described from the intraperitoneal administration of colloidal radioisotopes of gold ($^{198}$Au) and phosphorus ($^{32}$P), and cytotoxic drugs, and also from external irradiation of mediastinal and diaphragmatic lymphatics.

### Surgical relief

Patients with rapidly re-accumulating ascites who remain in reasonable general condition will often benefit from the insertion of a subcutaneous shunt joining the peritoneal cavity with the superior vena cava (LeVeen shunt). Insertion is relatively quick and simple but there is sometimes transient fever for a few days afterwards. There appear to be no problems arising from the shunting of neoplastic cells directly into the general circulation.

# Bowel Obstruction

The commonest cause of this type of obstruction in cancer patients is a primary bowel carcinoma, but it does occur quite frequently in patients with extensive intra-abdominal or pelvic tumour from any primary site. This is usually a terminal or immediately pre-terminal event but occasionally such obstruction may be due to tumour that is readily treatable, e.g. lymphoma. Other relevant causes include post-surgical or radiation adhesions, and radiation stricture.

The clinical diagnosis is based on manifestations such as nausea, vomiting, colic, constipation, distension and visible peristalsis and will be confirmed by an erect abdominal X-ray showing distended loops of bowel and multiple fluid levels. Initial therapy involves nasogastric suction and intravenous fluids which usually results in a substantial improvement in the patient's general condition. Surgical exploration is then indicated in patients without an established cause and without extensive untreatable malignancy. For patients with very advanced malignancy it is often possible to manage bowel obstruction conservatively with a low residue (mainly liquid) diet, anti-emetics, anti-spasmodics, analgesia and sedation as required. Surgery for the majority of these patients with an otherwise poor prognosis carries a high mortality, leaves them with a colostomy or ileostomy, adds very little if anything to the quality or quantity of life and should therefore be avoided if at all possible.

Conservative management is possible without intravenous fluids and nasogastric suction. Metoclopramide and domperidone should be avoided in these patients since small bowel motility may be increased and colic made worse. Useful anti-emetics include prochlorperazine or chlorpromazine (orally, by suppository or parenterally) or haloperidol (orally or parenterally). Loperamide 2 mg qds is useful for colic and hyoscine 0.3–0.6 mg sublingually prn can be helpful and may be taken before meals if food precipitates the colic. Persistent severe colic may require a hyoscine or atropine infusion, or a coeliac plexus block. Patients with incomplete obstruction may benefit from faecal softeners, e.g. docusate, Milpar or arachis oil retention enemas. Purgatives or high enemas should be avoided as they can worsen the colic.

# Brain Metastases

These are most common in patients with carcinomas of breast and bronchus, but can occur with almost any malignancy.

Common manifestations include personality change (sometimes very subtle), headache (usually due to raised intracranial pressure and worst on waking or changing posture), nausea and vomiting, fits and motor or sensory deficits. Papilloedema is relatively uncommon. The diagnosis is best confirmed by CT (or MRI) scan, but this is not always appropriate in the face of classical symptomatology in an already incurable patient.

Brain metastases are usually surrounded by some cerebral oedema and so there is often a dramatic short-term improvement with dexamethasone 4 mg tds-qds reducing if possible to a maintenance dose of, for example, 2 mg bd. Some patients benefit from a short course of cranial irradiation, especially those for whom high dose dexamethasone is ineffective or cannot be reduced. The duration of benefit however is usually only a small number of months, and alopecia is inevitable.

The blood-brain barrier is usually destroyed in brain metastases. Cytotoxic chemotherapy with drugs not normally thought capable of crossing it can therefore achieve useful palliation for some patients with relatively chemoresponsive malignancies.

A very small number of cancer patients develop an apparently solitary brain metastasis a long time (sometimes several years) after successful treatment for their primary tumour with no evidence of metastatic disease elsewhere. These may benefit substantially from surgical removal, perhaps followed by cranial irradiation, and such an approach can sometimes be curative.

# Pleural Effusion

This is very common, particularly in patients with carcinomas of bronchus, breast and ovary, and lymphomas. The effusion is almost always an exudate but cytology is quite often negative even when the cause is undoubtedly neoplastic, and particularly when it is due to lymphatic obstruction secondary to extensive mediastinal lymphadenopathy. However, it should never be forgotten that there may be a non-neoplastic cause for a cytologically negative effusion in a cancer patient, e.g. infection, infarction, heart failure and connective tissue disease; a pleural biopsy should be performed where there is doubt. Neoplastic effusions may be bilateral but are usually unilateral on the side of a causative lung carcinoma. Effusions from breast cancer are also more common on the side of the primary because of local spread via intercostal and ipselateral mediastinal lymphatics.

## Pleural aspiration

This is not necessary for all patients with effusions. In particular smaller effusions often cause no symptoms. Effusions do not necessarily increase in size and indeed they may regress as a result of successful systemic treatment.

No more than 1.5 litres (often ≤ 1 litre) should usually be aspirated on any one occasion. The removal of greater amounts (> 2 litres/24 hours) can cause pain and increased dyspnoea due to the precipitation of pulmonary oedema. In patients with bilateral effusions only one side should be aspirated on any one occasion. Aspiration of pleural effusions is a potentially hazardous procedure and should always be performed with great care. Adverse sequelae include pain, rupture of intercostal vessels and pneumothorax. More seriously, it can result in rupture of pulmonary vessels with massive haemoptysis, empyema and air embolism, and in penetration of the heart muscle or coronary vessels. The latter may result from cardiomegaly not previously visible on the chest X-ray because of a large left-sided effusion.

A chest X-ray should always be taken before an effusion is tapped. Prior to aspiration the patient should be positioned in a comfortable sitting position in bed. It is often helpful for the patient's forearms and elbows to be supported by a bed table fixed at the appropriate level. Aspiration must be a sterile procedure with gloves and mask being worn; pleural fluid is a good bacterial growth medium. The patient should be draped and the site of aspiration and surrounding skin thoroughly cleansed with cotton wool balls saturated in an antiseptic solution, moving outwards rather than inwards, in rotatory fashion. The patient should be told to report any pain during the aspiration and any feeling that he is about to cough.

Pleural aspiration should be done via a needle inserted perpendicular to the skin just above (not below) a rib margin, in order to lessen the risk of damage to an intercostal vessel. Prior to insertion the needle track should be infiltrated with 5–10 mls 1 per cent lignocaine. To help to ensure that the aspiration needle is inserted along the track that has been infiltrated with local anaesthetic, it is important that both needles are inserted slowly, gently and perpendicularly, aiming for the centre of the chest. A very small amount of pleural effusion should be withdrawn into the anaesthetic syringe, in order to confirm the position of the needle tip. The needle should then be very slightly withdrawn to a position where no further fluid can be sucked back and a generous further amount of local anaesthetic then injected. This will help to ensure adequate anaesthesia of the otherwise very sensitive parietal pleura. No further injection should take place as the needle is withdrawn as this can seed neoplastic cells and cause a subsequent troublesome superficial metastatic nodule.

A fairly wide bore needle should be used for the aspiration as this helps shorten the duration of the procedure, which is usually kinder and safer for the patient. The needle should never be inserted more than a very little way deeper in than the parietal pleura. It is reassuring if a very slight change in position of the needle during the procedure results in aspiration temporarily ceasing because the needle tip has moved outside the parietal pleura. Some method must be used to ensure that the needle cannot be accidentally pushed in further. This may be by positioning the other hand between the point of insertion and the syringe, or by binding a short length of adhesive tape around the needle. The needle must be withdrawn if the patient is about to cough or coughs, in order to reduce the risk of pneumothorax.

Sometimes aspiration proves difficult and this can be due to overestimation of the fluid component of radiological opacification, and to loculation. It is dangerous to push the needle in further and at different angles in the attempt to aspirate more fluid. When there is loculation an ultrasound scan may be helpful in indicating a potentially more fruitful site for aspiration.

A chest X-ray should be taken after each aspiration in order to assess the amount of residual fluid, show other previously obscured pathology, provide a base-line for comparison with later films and demonstrate any iatrogenic pneumothorax.

## Pleurodesis

Some patients require repeated pleural aspiration and can derive substantial benefit from a pleurodesis. This is the sealing together of the visceral and parietal pleura, thereby obliterating the potential space in which a pleural effusion may accumulate. The pleural effusion should first be aspirated to dryness in order to achieve approximation of the visceral and parietal pleura. This can only be achieved by the insertion of an intercostal underwater drain, with suction if necessary; the drain can be clamped in order to prevent too rapid drainage. Once drainage appears to be complete the drain should be left *in situ* for about 24 hours. It is then removed immediately after instillation of a small volume of a sclerosing agent which causes local inflammation, thereby encouraging the pleural layers to fuse. A variety of agents has been used; tetracycline 1 g in 50 ml normal saline, bleomycin 60 mg in 100 ml normal saline and freeze-dried *Corynebacterium parvum* 7 mg in 20 ml normal saline are all of established efficacy and relatively well tolerated. Tetracycline is probably the best tolerated and may produce more than a merely inflammatory effect: the oxidised drug has been shown to exert a cytostatic effect on tumour cells *in vitro*.

Some pain is very common after this procedure but, although it is usually transient and not severe, it is advisable to add 200 mg lignocaine, and essential to ensure adequate systemic analgesic medication. After instillation and removal of the drain the patient should then be encouraged to turn by 90° every 10 minutes for 40 minutes with the foot of the bed elevated, in order to help distribute the sclerosant over a wide area. C parvum and bleomycin can both cause fever. This technique prevents significant re-accumulation of fluid in about 75 per cent of patients.

Pleurectomy may be considered on extremely rare occasions for intractable effusion in patients in very good general health and with a very good prognosis. However, the risk of mortality from the procedure is about 10 per cent.

# Spinal Cord/Cauda Equina Compression

This is most common in patients with bronchial, breast and prostatic carcinoma but it can occur as a result of metastatic spread from almost any malignancy, including lymphomas and myeloma. It may be due to extradural tumour or occur as a result of vertebral collapse following metastatic osteolysis. The neurological sequelae may be due to direct damage to the spinal cord or to interference with its blood supply causing infarction; the latter is suggested when neurological deterioration is sudden. Cord compression usually produces fairly rapidly progressive symptoms and signs, but cauda equina compression (affecting lower motor neurones) is often a more indolent process.

It must not be forgotten that there are causes of paraparesis that do not involve spinal cord compression by tumour or collapsed bone. Previous moderate to high dose radiotherapy to the spinal cord, e.g. for carcinoma of bronchus or Hodgkin's disease, can cause a radiation myelitis. Very rarely a transverse myelitis occurs as a non-metastatic para-neoplastic phenomenon. Multiple sclerosis is another possibility and this can be aggravated by radiotherapy. For all these conditions radiotherapy for the presumed cord compression could be positively harmful.

## Assessment

Leg weakness is the commonest initial symptom of cord or cauda equina compression and must always be taken very seriously. Sensory disturbance is also very common and even when not volunteered or admitted sensation to pin-prick (very light pressure using a sterile needle) must be tested. A sensory level is often found and helps to localise the position of the lesion. It must not be forgotten that there is a discrepancy between any vertebra and the corresponding dermatome of approximately 1 in the cervical spine, 2 in the thoracic spine and 3 in the lumbar spine. For example, a sensory level at the T10 dermatome (level of umbilicus) may occur with a lesion at the level of the 8th thoracic vertebra. Loss of pelvic visceral sensation and sphincter control is also common, but commonly follows weakness and disturbance of skin sensation. In addition to assessment of power and skin sensation, all patients should be tested for altered tone, sustained clonus, and abnormalities of tendon, plantar and anal reflexes. Back pain and localised tenderness to mild percussion are both very common in patients with vertebral metastasis.

Ideally neurological compression and the exact level of the pathology should be determined by myelography, but waiting for this to be done can take time and often the clinical and plain film findings provide extremely strong circumstantial evidence. Plain films will frequently show evidence of any vertebral pathology, and will also sometimes show a soft tissue mass.

## Treatment

The possibility of cord or cauda equina compression must always be taken very seriously since very prompt treatment, particularly for cord compression, may substantially influence the neurological outcome; even hours can be crucial. Immediate intervention can prevent further neurological deterioration and sometimes there is substantial or complete recovery. The chance of recovery of mobility is inversely related to the degree of initial impairment. Although many of these patients have incurable disease many would normally be expected to live for at least several months, and therefore retention of mobility, sphincter control and independence is of great importance to the quality of their remaining life. Management will be dependent on the length of the history, the nature of the neoplasm, the extent of the disease, the prognosis and the severity of the neurological disturbance. The chance of any recovery for patients with complete paraplegia is always extremely low.

High dose dexamethasone, 4 mg qds, is justified immediately for almost all patients in an attempt to lessen any possible component of oedema causing pressure, but the important decision for many patients concerns whether or not to offer surgical decompression. It is usually helpful to discuss the situation immediately with a neurosurgeon, or orthopaedic surgeon with relevant expertise. Patients in good general condition with a reasonable prognosis, short history, no marked vertebral collapse and only partial loss of power are often considered particularly suitable for surgery, particularly if there is no widespread metastatic disease. Surgery is also usually indicated when this is the first manifestation of possible malignancy, and may be the only way of establishing the diagnosis. Myelography is essential prior to surgery. Both posterior and anterior (trans-abdominal) surgical approaches are used, depending on the position of the compression.

Surgery is undoubtedly the quickest way of relieving compression, but sadly a complication for a minority is exacerbation of the neurological deficit, often with complete paraplegia. For most patients not considered suitable for surgery immediate palliative radiotherapy is appropriate, usually over 1–2 weeks. Radiotherapy is also considered the treatment of choice for highly radioresponsive neoplasms, particularly lymphomas, myeloma and small cell carcinoma of bronchus. It is reasonable to continue the dexamethasone for the duration of radiotherapy but it should be stopped or very rapidly tailed off subsequently: a steroid myopathy will worsen the weakness.

*Supportive care*

Sadly many patients make minimal neurological recovery, or none at all, and thus supportive care becomes very important. This involves not only the provision of personnel, e.g. home helps, district nurses to help with bathing, but also advice and its implementation concerning alterations at home, e.g. ramps for the wheel chair, rails on the lavatory walls, bed hoists and the fitting of a downstairs bathroom. The involvement of the medical social worker and occupational therapist is usually invaluable.

# Superior Vena Caval Obstruction

The commonest cause by far is mediastinal spread from lung cancer. Non-Hodgkin's lymphoma is the next most common cause and occasionally it can occur as a result of extensive mediastinal lymphadenopathy from other tumours, e.g. teratoma, breast carcinoma. Very rarely it is due to a nonmalignant cause such as large retrosternal goitre or aortic aneurysm.

## Manifestations

The signs of superior vena caval obstruction include distended neck veins, swollen and plethoric face, neck and arms, dyspnoea, prominent veins over the chest with often a characteristic 'flare' of very small veins under the breasts (males and females), and occasionally raised intracranial pressure with headache and papilloedema. This is often the first manifestation of malignancy and these patients should be carefully palpated for readily accessible tumour, especially in the supraclavicular fossae, since this may enable a tissue diagnosis; palpation here is often difficult however because of the swelling. These patients should be carefully examined for lymphadenopathy elsewhere or splenomegaly, in order to exclude the possibility of lymphoma. This should especially be considered in those who have not smoked.

## Investigations

The chest X-ray will usually show a large mediastinal mass. Sometimes there will be a separate, more peripheral, mass strongly suggestive of a primary lung carcinoma. Sputum should be sent for cytology and a fine needle aspirate taken from any palpable tumour. More invasive procedures such as bronchoscopic biopsy and mediastinoscopy are hazardous because of the risk of haemorrhage and it is usually considered justifiable to proceed very promptly to treatment without a tissue diagnosis, in view of the extremely high probability of a malignant cause and the distressing and potentially fatal nature of the syndrome. Also, the longer the duration of the obstruction the greater the likelihood of secondary thrombosis which may cause permanent obstruction even when there has been a satisfactory tumour response. However, it should be documented that there is a possibility of lymphoma in patients without a tissue diagnosis, since this has important implications for subsequent management. This possibility is increased if there is rapid and substantial regression of a mediastinal mass with palliative radiotherapy.

## *Treatment*

Patients with respiratory embarrassment should be offered supplemental oxygen. Dexamethasone 4 mg tds-qds for a week or so is justifiable in an attempt to lessen any oedematous component. A short course of palliative radiotherapy is the oncological treatment of choice for most patients. If this cannot be arranged promptly, or if there are features suggestive of a lymphoma or small cell bronchial carcinoma, or if one of these diagnoses is established, cytotoxic chemotherapy may be used. Bolus injections of cytotoxic drugs should not be given into an arm in which the veins do not collapse on elevation, since this carries a risk of local drug stasis and severe thrombophlebitis.

**NOTES**

**NOTES**

# CHAPTER 15

# Aspects of Physical Rehabilitation

For many patients treatment for cancer, even when it has been curative, is followed by major problems, both psychological and physical. Successful rehabilitation can therefore profoundly improve their quality of life. In this chapter some of the more common sequelae of treatment are briefly discussed. There is quite a large number of organisations and groups which can provide valuable help to patients with specific problems, and some of those found in Britain are listed at the end of the book.

## Colostomy

Modern colostomy management usually succeeds in avoiding the discomfort, embarrassment and social isolation that used to occur from unpleasant smells, leakage and skin soreness. Patients can now lead almost normal lives, including swimming, if desired. Patients should have their misapprehensions corrected if possible and be fully informed about all practical aspects as long as possible before surgery. Potential difficulties such as impaired vision or manual dexterity should be identified. Patients with a history of allergic skin disease can develop reactions to the bag adhesive and patch testing is therefore advisable. Many hospitals enjoy the extremely useful services of a stoma-care nurse who can do much to minimise both physical and psychological difficulties.

The more distal the site of the colostomy the greater the absorption of water and the more formed the stool: a caecostomy discharges very irritating liquid stools. There are two types of bag or pouch in use: a drainable one for use when the stools are semi-solid or liquid, and a closed one for formed stools. There are also two types of colostomy appliance: a one-piece appliance where the protective skin barrier and the bag or pouch are integral and which attaches straight to the skin, and a two-piece appliance in which a separate bag is clipped securely on to a separate protective skin barrier around the stoma. These bags can be changed very easily without disturbing the skin or stoma, and the separate skin barrier needs to be changed only every 3–5 days.

Stoma sizes vary considerably and can also shrink in the months after surgery. An ill-fitting appliance not only feels uncomfortable but it may also leak or cause irritation and soreness. For some patients it is convenient to evacuate the bowel by irrigation daily or every other day, with the aim of preventing spontaneous evacuation with may occur at any time. However, this usually takes 30–45 minutes and is not always feasible for frail and elderly patients because they can find the procedure exhausting or because they would be dependent on someone else to do it. Irrigation usually prevents constipation or faecal impaction, but for others a good fluid and dietary fibre intake is important. Bulk-forming laxatives are often helpful. Most patients can continue with their previous diet but peas, beans and fizzy drinks can cause excessive flatus. Another cause of this is excessive ingestion of air, which may occur in anxious patients, in those who smoke, chew gum, chew with an open mouth and talk while eating. Flatus also tends to be increased during air travel and when the bowel is empty: unhurried regular meals are advisable. Flatus filters are now available with some colostomy pouches.

The ingestion of cabbage, baked beans, onions, eggs, fish, highly spiced foods, curries and alcohol tends to increase unpleasant odours but yoghurt and buttermilk may reduce them. However, the proper management of modern appliances should ensure no escaping gas except when the bag is emptied or the colostomy irrigated.

Dermatitis can be caused by diarrhoea, leakage, candida,

contact dermatitis and cytotoxic chemotherapy or local radiotherapy. Leakage is usually the result of a poorly fitting appliance. Candidal infection should be treated by applying nystatin powder at each change – ointment prevents adherence, as do any other greasy substances (e.g. barrier or antiseptic creams) or solutions. Other sites may be the source of the infection and should be identified and treated.

# Dental Damage

Specialised dental care is particularly important in the management of patients who are to have, or have had, extensive orofacial radiotherapy. Radiotherapy causes mucositis which usually subsides over two to three weeks (see section on stomatitis) and can also cause impaired or altered taste which may last for many months or even years. However, of perhaps equal importance to patients who have retained their own teeth is the impact of treatment on tooth and gum disease.

Radiation damages the minor and major salivary glands. Patients with advanced tumours in the mouth or pharynx, or patients having wide field radiotherapy for Hodgkin's disease often receive irradiation to parotid and submandibular salivary glands on both sides. This produces a dry mouth, which many patients find extremely unpleasant, and which only recovers slowly and partially with time; in addition there is a qualitative saliva change. These effects render the mouth extremely prone to severe gum disease and caries. In turn this can predispose to the development of osteoradionecrosis of the mandible, fortunately now a rare complication.

It is important to get an expert assessment of the status of gums and teeth prior to treatment. Appropriate conservative or extractive dental care can then be given and the patients advised on the importance of meticulous long-term attention to oral and dental hygiene. Many patients derive symptomatic benefit from the prescription of aerosol sprays of artificial saliva.

# Ileal Conduit

This is the commonest type of permanent urinary diversion. The ureters are transplanted into a length of isolated ileum, one end of which is brought to the surface as a stoma. The length of ileum does not act as a reservoir: urine seeps continuously from the stoma. As with other stomas skin irritation can occur, but here the fitting of the appliance is even more critical if leakage is to be prevented. Disposable and semi-disposable appliances are available. The latter consists of a re-usable faceplate or gasket to which is attached a disposable single-use pouch. As with other ostomies a virtually normal life is now feasible with modern appliances.

Meticulous hygiene is important in order to prevent urinary tract infection. Infection may be suggested by the urine's appearance or smell. Bacteriological confirmation should be on a specimen obtained by catheterisation of the conduit and not from the pouch, thus avoiding contamination. Patients should be encouraged to report any urinary or stomal symptoms promptly and renal function should be checked at least annually. The urine will normally contain some mucus; this is a secretion from the ileal mucosa.

Good fluid intake is important and normal urinary odour can be lessened by fruit juices, which make it more acidic. Warm water is usually sufficient to remove the appliance adhesive as soaps and solvents can cause skin sensitisation. Skin soreness may also be avoided by very gentle removal of the appliance.

# Lymphoedema

Lymphoedema can be one of the most upsetting of cancer-related problems. It can be severe and disabling and is quite often present for the long remainder of the life of a cured patient. It is most commonly seen in the arm after treatment for breast cancer and may be caused by metastatic lymphadenopathy although it is more often iatrogenic. Both surgery and radiotherapy can cause it independently but the combination of the two, particularly when there has been an axillary dissection, is particularly predisposing. Late onset lymphoedema is more likely to be due to recurrent tumour but iatrogenesis remains a possibility.

For patients with mild lymphoedema usually only some explanation and reassurance is needed; for others a variety of measures may be tried. Useful elevation of the arm is rarely feasible but may be worth trying, particularly raising the arm in a sling or on pillows above heart level at night. Isometric arm muscle exercise with the limb elevated helps some patients by activating the muscle pump. Patients should also be encouraged to wear a good-quality arm stocking and tight elastic glove. It is also worth trying an intermittent pneumatic compression cuff. This gives some benefit of very variable magnitude in about 50 per cent of patients. Any improvement is usually apparent within a month of starting treatment, but further reduction in girth is unlikely after four months. If pneumatic compression is successful it needs to be repeated regularly, and it may then be worth while for the patients to buy their own pump. It is time consuming – at least a couple of hours a day are usually required.

Some patients may derive benefit, possibly of both a physical and a psychological nature, from a manual methodical squeezing of the arm progressively upwards, performed by their spouse. Diuretics are rarely helpful and should certainly not be prescribed on a long-term basis unless there is clear objective evidence of efficacy, as judged by circumferential measurement. Very occasionally surgery may be considered for patients with gross oedema. In Homan's operation the oedematous tissues are excised: the medial side of the arm and forearm first, followed by the lateral side about three months later. However, this procedure does not benefit hand oedema.

Lymphoedematous limbs are particularly prone to widespread cellulitis after only a slight infected injury. When gardening or doing other similar jobs a protective glove must be worn. Thimbles should be worn when sewing, and fiddling with nail cuticles or finger biting avoided. No injections should be given in an affected arm and antibiotic treatment is indicated at the earliest evidence of infection anywhere on the affected limb. Rings can cut into oedematous fingers and it may be advisable to remove them, by cutting off if necessary. The affected arm should not be used for carrying anything heavy. Lymphoedema in the leg(s) of a cancer patient is usually due to tumour. Appropriate oncological treatment may occasionally relieve it, but in most patients it is persistent. Elevation of the legs whenever possible can sometimes help, as may the wearing of tight elastic stockings.

Lymphoedema in the submandibular region is a not uncommon side effect of radical neck irradiation. There is a bilateral and symmetrical boggy swelling (dewlap) which can cause the patient considerable anxiety as he may think that it represents recurrent tumour. Fortunately it usually subsides gradually with time.

# Mastectomy

Mastectomy should be performed only as an elective procedure, with the patient prepared as far as possible beforehand. Many hospitals now have breast care nurses who see patients before and after surgery, advise on physical and cosmetic rehabilitation, and who can substantially reduce both physical and psychological morbidity.

The now infrequently performed standard radical mastectomy involves removal of both pectoralis major and minor muscles, with consequent reduced shoulder strength. Lesser operations do not usually cause significant weakness but nevertheless mobility is inevitably impaired after surgery, particularly in those who have had surgery to the axilla. A vigorous exercise programme after surgery is important to the rapid restoration of normal mobility and prevention, or treatment, of stiffness. Active shoulder exercises should be in progress by five or six days after surgery, but they should avoid excessive tension across suture lines and satisfactory wound healing should be ascertained first. Following suture removal, daily active exercises should be performed with the aim of rapidly re-establishing the normal complete range of movement (flexion, extension, abduction and internal and external rotation).

Cosmetic rehabilitation usually involves the provision of a

temporary prosthesis very soon after the operation, and a symmetrical and comfortable permanent prosthesis as soon as possible – these are most commonly liquid silicone or foam filled. Some women request a reconstructive surgical procedure, which commonly involves a silastic gel implant with or without a latissimus dorsi or other flap. This is usually feasible, but probably best delayed until a few months after mastectomy and after any adjuvant radiotherapy or cytotoxic chemotherapy.

For many women the loss of a breast adds substantially to the psychological morbidity arising from the diagnosis of breast cancer. In particular it causes difficulties with body image and libido, thereby adding to anxiety and depression. Some benefit may be gained from counselling, psychotropic medication and specialised psychiatric assistance. (See chapter on psychological support and sections on lymphoedema and sex life.)

# Nutrition

Poor nutrition is an extremely common problem in cancer patients, affecting almost all in the terminal stages. Although this is often a major cause of weight loss, the latter is quite often seen in those who have maintained a normal nutritional intake. This is due to diversion of protein and calories to the tumour and to humorally mediated metabolic disturbances exerted by the tumour. Muscle wasting is a prominent feature of cancer cachexia. In these patients attempts to increase food intake do not result in significant weight gain.

Poor nutrition impairs the body's tolerance to surgery, radiotherapy and cytotoxic chemotherapy, and recovery after treatment. Vigorous measures to increase or maintain nutrition may therefore sometimes be indicated in patients who are to receive, or have just received, potentially curative treatment. These may include intravenous total parenteral nutrition and, often in patients with severe radiation mucositis from treatment to the head and neck, fine bore nasogastric tube feeding. The majority of patients who have received, or are receiving, potentially curative treatments satisfactorily manage to maintain as near to normal nutrition as is possible when given help and advice. The emphasis should be on maximising protein and calorie intake; manoeuvres such as the addition of eggs to beverages, ice-cream to desserts and preparing powdered soups with milk may help. Patients who have enjoyed beer or wine in the past should be encouraged to drink them as they are a good source of calories and can improve morale. A variety of liquid food supplements are available and some have a variety of flavourings; experimentation is often helpful. For the majority of malnourished patients who have advanced, incurable disease vigorous attempts to increase protein and calorie intake are not justified.

In some situations dietary modification is appropriate. Patients receiving head and neck radiotherapy will find bland sloppy foods easier to ingest and hot, irritant foods should be avoided. A low-residue diet with minimal fruit intake will help to lessen diarrhoea in patients receiving abdominal or pelvic radiotherapy. Patients with the dumping syndrome or steatorrhoea after gastrectomy will benefit from reduced carbohydrate and fat intakes respectively.

Clinically overt vitamin or iron deficiency is unusual, but glossitis and angular cheilitis may be suggestive of this. Some patients whose nutritional intake is clearly deficient may benefit from multivitamin supplementation, however, if the patient is taking a normal balanced diet there is no proven benefit from vitamin or trace metal supplementation. Patients who have undergone gastrectomy should have vitamin B12 supplementation and these patients may also occasionally eventually develop osteomalacia. Abdominal or pelvic radiotherapy can occasionally cause malabsorption and B12 deficiency. It is possible that unnecessary folate supplementation may have a stimulatory effect on some cancers. (See section on anorexia.)

# Sex Life

Up to one third of patients with certain cancers may experience loss of sexual desire, impotence or inability to achieve orgasm. This is especially the case when body image is substantially impaired by mastectomy or colostomy, or even temporarily from chemotherapy-induced alopecia. The psychosocial and sexual impact of mutilating surgery is likely to be even more profound in the young, unmarried or divorced woman who would like to find a husband. Where it is technically feasible many women may benefit from reconstructive surgery.

Endocrine mechanisms can be involved in sexual dysfunction. Cytotoxic chemotherapy and radiotherapy can ablate ovarian hormonal secretion and, to a lesser extent, interfere with testicular hormonal production. Men with prostatic cancer may be treated by orchidectomy or hormone supplements and some can find gynaecomastia particularly disturbing. This can be prevented in the majority of patients by a single high dose superficial radiation treatment to each breast before hormonal manipulation.

For other patients there may be mechanical or neurological reasons for sexual dysfunction, as a result of pelvic surgery or radiotherapy. Radical bladder, prostatic and rectal surgery carries a very high risk of autonomic neurological damage resulting in impotence, and to a lesser extent pelvic radiotherapy can do the same. In other patients surgery to the bladder neck or a retroperitoneal lymphadenectomy may result not in impotence but in retrograde ejaculation or a failure of ejaculation. Radical hysterectomy results in a shortening of the vagina, and pelvic radiotherapy (particularly intracavitary) results in greatly diminished vaginal secretions and a tendency for the vagina to seal off if not kept patent.

It is important to consider the overall sexuality and psychological status of the patient rather than merely the physical dysfunction complained of. Patients may feel unclean and that their cancer is infectious, a venereal disease, or a punishment for past sexual behaviour. They may feel that it is not right to enter into sexual activity whilst they are ill, for fear that it may sap their strength. One partner may assume more of a parental than sexually partnering rôle. For some the whole burden may threaten a marital relationship although for others, particularly those whose relationship and communication was previously very strong, the whole experience may bring them even closer together. (See chapter on psychological support.) A variety of psychological techniques is available to help rehabilitation, where appropriate, for a persistent problem. These are usually best undertaken by a suitably experienced clinical psychologist or psychiatrist. However, many patients may benefit merely from being told that they can or should resume sexual activity, although it is usually up to the doctor to bring the subject up.

After pelvic radiotherapy in previously sexually active women it is particularly important to advise the resumption of intercourse as soon as the acute reaction has subsided, otherwise vaginal adhesions will develop. Lubricating jelly is often necessary and patients should be warned that initially it may be uncomfortable or painful but that this will improve with time. They should also be warned that it may cause slight vaginal bleeding if there is any vaginal telangiectasia, a not uncommon occurrence after radiotherapy. For women without a sexual partner it is often reasonable to suggest that they keep the vagina patent by inserting a dilator (or candle) regularly. The prevention of adhesions will allow examination of the vaginal vault at follow-up and may thus enable early detection of recurrence. Some patients can benefit from penile prosthetic surgery or vaginal reconstruction.

# Tracheostomy

Loss of a larynx is a devastating psychosocial blow. Usually an attempt is made to train patients to develop oesophageal speech. The aim is to trap air in the oesophagus and to release it upwards in a controlled manner so as to cause vibration in the pharyngo-oesophageal sphincter. The voice produced in some patients can resemble laryngeal phonation to a remarkable extent, but unfortunately only about one third of patients manage to develop good oesophageal speech. Difficulty may occur as a result of surgical deformity or nerve damage, radiation damage, deafness and lack of motivation. Some patients swallow air and develop distension and flatulence. If a pharyngectomy has been performed as well, then oesophageal speech will be impossible.

Various operations have been devised to produce a small

fistula between the trachea and oesophagus, thereby facili-
tating oesophageal speech by exhaling when the tracheostomy is occluded by a finger or valve sensitive to the increased
pressure required for speech. Although such procedures work
well in some patients, in others there are problems due to
aspiration of food where the fistula is too large, or due to the
fistula being too tight.

For many patients the best option may be the use of an
electrolarynx, a battery-powered device which emits a sound
of frequency comparable to normal speaking voice, which can
be applied to the tissues of the upper neck. Articulation in the
usual way then produces intelligible speech.

**NOTES**

# PART II

# Notes on the More Common Cancers

# CHAPTER 16

# Bladder Carcinoma

There are approximately 18 new cases annually per 100,000 population and the male/female ratio is 3:1. Over 90 per cent of bladder carcinomas are transitional cell carcinomas, arising from the normal urothelial lining. This can occasionally transform to a squamous epithelium under the influence of chronic irritation, and most of the remaining neoplasms are squamous carcinomas. Bladder neoplasia is more often characterised by a continuous spectrum between benign and malignant behaviour (with a tendency for the former to precede the latter, often by several years), than neoplasia in most other organs. This has led to a reluctance to classify any superficial tumour as benign.

Histologically benign, non-invasive urothelial papillomas have a recurrence rate of up to 50 per cent. About 20 per cent of patients with these tumours subsequently develop invasive carcinoma: this chance increases if there are multiple papillomas, which is often the case. Non-invasive neoplastic change can occur without exophytic growth: the presence of anaplastic cells within the confines of the urothelium is termed carcinoma-in-situ. These lesions may be roughened, thickened or haemorrhagic, but are essentially flat. Multicentric change, recurrence and the development of invasive carcinoma are again common.

Invasion through the basement membrane is first to the lamina propria, then to superficial and deep muscle, perivesical fat and adjacent organs. The propensity for invasion is closely related to the degree of differentiation. The outlook for patients with 'low grade' tumours is much better than for those with 'high grade' tumours.

The relative five-year survival rate for all bladder neoplasia, including non-invasive disease, is approximately 60 per cent, but for patients with non-invasive papillomas it is approximately 90 per cent, falling to 70 per cent at 10 years. The prognosis is even better for those with solitary papillomas, but substantially worse for those with carcinoma-in-situ, which has about a 35 per cent mortality rate at five years. Approximately 50 per cent of patients with very superficial invasion are cured, but when there is muscle invasion the chance of cure falls to 30 per cent and to below 10 per cent when there is extension outside the bladder. The outlook is better for younger patients and women, but worse for those with squamous carcinomas.

### Risk factors

Smoking; industrial exposure to aniline dyes, rubber, leather, paint, magenta, auramine, benzidine, naphthylamine, naphthylthiourea (pesticide) and other organic chemicals; cyclophosphamide; schistosomiasis (squamous tumours).

### Spread

Metastases are rare with tumours that are only superficially invasive, but are present in 40 per cent of deeply invasive cases. Lymphatic spread occurs to pelvic lymph nodes and blood-borne spread principally to lung, liver and bones.

### Symptoms and signs

Haematuria
Frequency
Dysuria
Pain
Supraclavicular lymphadenopathy
Urethral nodularity
Pelvic mass
Leg oedema

# Treatment

## Radical

### Surgery

Transurethral resection or diathermy is the mainstay of management of non-invasive tumours. Laser treatment is now under evaluation. The recurrence rate is, however, high and regular cystoscopy is essential. Intravesical chemotherapy or BCG can lower the rate of recurrence (see below). Transurethral resection is also appropriate for most patients with minimal invasion (of the lamina propria), but with no evidence of muscle involvement.

Although bladder carcinoma has a strong tendency towards multicentricity, partial cystectomy may be appropriate for carefully selected patients with small solitary invasive carcinomas when there is no evidence of mucosal instability elsewhere. Total cystectomy is indicated for patients with both uncontrolled carcinoma-in-situ and papillomatosis, both of which are relatively radioresistant. It is an alternative to radiotherapy for tumours which invade muscle but which do not extend outside the bladder. Since the cure rates from the two modalities are comparable, cystectomy is often preferred as a salvage treatment following failure of radiotherapy.

Total cystectomy may be simple or radical, the latter involving removal of perivesical tissue, seminal vesicles and prostate or uterus and ovaries, plus or minus pelvic lymphadenectomy. The radical operation is generally preferred because of the increased margin of excision, although male impotence is inevitable. Urinary diversion is usually achieved with an ileal conduit, opening on the lower abdominal wall. The conduit should be short, and should not act as a repository for urine since absorption can cause electrolytic disturbance. (See chapters on rehabilitation and psychological support.)

### Radiotherapy

Radiotherapy is usually given with megavoltage teletherapy but interstitial implants are also sometimes used for the treatment of small tumours. Radical radiotherapy is not usually considered justified for growths extending outside the bladder, or for the elderly.

The acute side effects of radical radiotherapy include frequency and diarrhoea, but these are not usually severe. Late complications include fibrosis causing a contracted bladder and/or 'frozen pelvis', bowel damage and bleeding from bladder telangiectasia. (See section on haemorrhage in Chapter 10 in Part I.) The irradiated bladder is also susceptible to infection and ulceration.

### Combined modality

There is some evidence to suggest that the combination of pre-operative, sub-radical dosage, pelvic radiotherapy and cystectomy may lead to a higher cure rate than radiotherapy alone. It is given principally with the aim of sterilising any involved pelvic lymph nodes.

### Cytotoxic chemotherapy

Trials of adjuvant systemic cytotoxic chemotherapy are in progress but as yet there is no evidence that this can improve the long-term outlook.

Courses of intravesical instillations of cytotoxic drugs, usually administered weekly or monthly for three to six months, have been shown to suppress the recurrence of superficial growths. Patients with multiple lesions and a history of recurrence are particularly suitable for such treatment. Although there is some evidence that intravesical chemotherapy may reduce the likelihood of invasive cancer, it has not yet been established that it can improve the chance of long-term survival.

### BCG

Intravesical BCG has been shown to have comparable or even greater efficacy than intravesical cytotoxic chemotherapy in reducing the recurrence of superficial tumours, and it is particularly useful in patients with carcinoma-in-situ; it can however cause troublesome cystitis.

## Palliative

### Surgery

Haematuria may sometimes be controlled by diathermy, cryosurgery, or hydrostatic pressure (inflating a balloon within the bladder). Internal iliac artery embolisation will usually control severe bleeding.

### Radiotherapy

This is usually the preferred palliative treatment. A relatively low dose given over a couple of weeks will control haematuria in the great majority of patients. This treatment is usually well tolerated although some minor bowel disturbance is common.

### Chemotherapy

About one third of patients will respond to drugs such as cisplatinum and methotrexate given systemically as single agents, and more than 50 per cent to some combinations of drugs. However, as most remissions do not last more than a few months it is debatable whether the toxicity justifies the frequent use of chemotherapy for palliation.

### Tranexamic acid

This anti-fibrinolytic drug can sometimes be helpful in controlling haematuria, although there is a risk of clot retention; a lower dose should be used where there is renal impairment. This drug should not be used if there is a history of thrombo-embolic disease.

### Follow-up

Regular cystoscopic follow-up is essential after treatment for superficial neoplasia, and after any radical treatment for invasive carcinoma not involving total cystectomy. There is no point in subjecting patients to routine cystoscopy after palliative treatment.

## Practice points

1 A thorough industrial history is important: patients or their families may be entitled to compensation.
2 Clinical examination should include palpation of the supraclavicular fossae and urethra. Urethral nodularity may be the only evidence of extra-vesical tumour.

## NOTES

# CHAPTER 17

# Brain Tumours

The annual incidence of primary brain tumours is approximately five per 100,000 population, and the male/female ratio is 3:2. The majority of adult brain tumours arise from glial cells and are known as gliomas, but about 15 per cent arise from the meninges (meningiomas). The majority of adult tumours are situated supratentorially, contrasting with the largely infratentorial position in children, in whom brain tumours are proportionally much more common. In adults the majority of all brain tumours are metastases, but this chapter is concerned only with primary tumours.

The majority of gliomas arise from astrocytes, the supporting cells for neurones. Astrocytomas vary substantially in their malignancy, and may be classified as 'low-grade' or 'high-grade' tumours. They are usually aggressive tumours showing frequent mitoses, pleomorphism and a tendency to infiltrate widely, often far more extensively than is apparent radiologically or macroscopically. The most malignant type is sometimes referred to as *glioblastoma multiforme*.

Oligodendrogliomas in contrast are more often relatively benign, discrete and slow growing. Pure oligodendroglioma is however rare, and these tumours may be 'mixed' with other malignant glial elements: the prognosis is determined by the most malignant elements. Ependymomas, derived from the ciliated cells lining the ventricles, are usually intermediate in malignancy but can disseminate widely via the CSF; this occurs particularly in the higher-grade tumours. Medullo-blastomas arise from primitive neuroepithelial cells in the roof of the fourth ventricle. These tumours occasionally occur in young adults but are usually tumours of childhood and adolescence. They too have a tendency to spread via the CSF. Primary brain lymphomas are always high-grade aggressive neoplasms. Nearly all meningiomas are slow-growing and histologically benign.

Although some tumours are slow growing and histologically at the benign end of the spectrum, they may nevertheless be malignant in their effects by virtue of their position and ability to interfere with normal neurological function. Very small tumours in certain situations may produce devastating effects, for example by causing obstructive hydrocephalus, whilst it is often surprising that other much larger tumours do not disrupt normal function to a far greater extent. Metastatic spread outside the CNS is extremely rare for all tumours.

The two-year survival of patients with the common aggressive astrocytomas is only around 5–10 per cent, and very, very few are cured. For lower-grade astrocytomas, ependymomas and medulloblastomas the five-year survival rates approach 50 per cent and are higher still for patients with oligodendrogliomas and meningiomas. Although not all five-year survivors will be cured, some patients with the most indolent neoplasms, particularly meningiomas, will have a normal life expectancy.

## Risk factors

Ionising radiation; neurofibromatosis (gliomas); immunosuppression, particularly following organ transplantation and with AIDS (lymphomas).

## Symptoms and signs

Headache (often worst on waking)
Epilepsy
Mental or personality change
Nausea/vomiting
Long tract/cranial nerve disturbance
Papilloedema
Drowsiness/coma

# Management

## Radical

### Surgery

Radical surgery by itself is curative for some patients with relatively localised and accessible neoplasms, particularly meningiomas, low-grade astrocytomas and pure oligodendrogliomas. Reliance on the appearances on a CT scan for the diagnosis of primary brain malignancy means that in approximately five per cent of cases a non-malignant or potentially curable lesion such as an abscess or meningioma will be missed. Therefore, although biopsy carries its own risks, it is usually attempted except in the case of neoplasms of the brain stem and other surgically 'inaccessible' sites. MRI scanning does however offer the prospect of more accurate radiological diagnosis.

For many patients the position and extent of the tumour precludes radical removal. Where possible, however, a substantial debulking of the tumour may sometimes provide symptomatic improvement, and for a few patients it will contribute to ultimate eradication. Such debulking may relieve internal hydrocephalus, but quite often this requires surgical attention prior to definitive treatment; ventricular drainage and relief of pressure is achieved by the insertion of a ventriculo-atrial or ventriculo-peritoneal shunt. For some neoplasms this carries a remote risk of systemic dissemination and ideally a cell filter should be incorporated.

Surgery should be preceded by a thorough medical assessment including that of lung, renal and clotting function. (Retained carbon dioxide can raise intracranial pressure.) Restriction of intra-operative fluid intake and the use of osmotic diuretics may be required to lessen cerebral oedema. Hypertension during surgery also increases cerebral oedema and sometimes surgery is therefore performed under controlled hypotension. As a prophylaxis against oedema dexamethasone should be administered for at least two days prior to surgery, and consideration should also be given to a prophylactic anticonvulsant. An anti-bacterial shampoo should be used on the preceding one or two days.

Very close monitoring is required after craniotomy, with frequent checking of neurological status and vital signs, especially pulse rate, blood pressure and appearance of the pupils. Fluids should be restricted and steroids and anti-convulsants continued. Anticoagulants are contra-indicated.

Complications of surgery include transient or permanent neurological deficit due to neuronal damage, oedema, cere-bro-vascular accident, haematoma, hydrocephalus and infection.

## Radiotherapy

Medulloblastomas, brain stem gliomas and ependymomas are moderately radiosensitive, and for these radiotherapy may often make the greatest (and sometimes the only) contribution to cure. For tumours with a propensity to dissemination via the CSF, particularly medulloblastomas and high-grade ependymomas, adjuvant irradiation of the whole 'cra-nio-spinal axis' improves the chance of cure. Radiotherapy is also the principal treatment modality for lymphomas but, when compared with the response to radiotherapy for local-ised lymphoma at other sites, the results are very disappoint-ing. For the common cerebral astrocytomas radiotherapy can prolong survival after surgery and for a small minority, chiefly those with lower-grade tumours, it may contribute to ultimate cure.

Cranial radiotherapy is usually well tolerated symptomati-cally. Alopecia is inevitable. Some radiation-induced or -ex-acerbated oedema is probably fairly common and it may cause nausea and vomiting, headache and drowsiness, but these symptoms usually respond to dexamethasone. High radiation doses carry a risk of late brain necrosis. There is some evi-dence to suggest that the risk of this is lower if relatively small individual daily doses are used; treatment courses therefore often last five to six weeks and sometimes longer.

## Cytotoxic chemotherapy

In the past it was thought that most cytotoxic drugs did not have the ability to enter brain tumours in useful concentrations because of the blood-brain barrier, however, this supposed barrier does not in fact exist for many tumours. Certain lipid soluble drugs do have the ability to penetrate this barrier, where it exists, and it is these that have been most investigated in the treatment of primary brain tumours, particularly the nitrosoureas (BCNU and CCNU), and procarbazine. Unfortunately the results are very disappointing: some randomised studies have demonstrated a slight increase in median survival from the addition of chemotherapy, but they do not appear to improve the chance of ultimate cure.

## Palliation

### Surgery

Relief of obstructive hydrocephalus by the insertion of ventriculo-atrial or ventriculo-peritoneal shunts can afford rapid symptom relief.

### Radiotherapy

Although radiotherapy is most commonly given with radical intent, any derived benefit is usually of a palliative nature. Sometimes quite remarkable short-term neurological improvement is seen during or following treatment for incurable tumours.

### Cytotoxic chemotherapy

About one third of patients with high-grade gliomas show an objective response to chemotherapy with drugs such as BCNU, CCNU, procarbazine and vincristine. However, the responses are usually short-lived and occur predominantly in patients with relatively well-differentiated tumours.

### Steroids

These have a very important rôle in palliation. Most advanced tumours have some intrinsic and surrounding oedema which usually responds well to high dose steroids, e.g. dexamethasone 4 mg tds or qds. The symptomatic improvement is usual-

ly rapid. Quite often this dose can subsequently be substantially reduced, e.g. to 2 mg bd, and an attempt to reduce the
dose should be made in view of the Cushingoid and myopathic
side effects.

## Other agents

Cerebral oedema sometimes causes rapid deterioration,
which may require equally rapid correction. The osmotic
dehydrating agents mannitol or urea, administered intravenously, produce a quick diuresis with usually an early
clinical improvement. For mannitol the adult dose is 1 litre of
20 per cent solution over 24 hours. Contra-indications include
congestive cardiac failure, renal failure, and hepatic failure
for urea.

## Follow-up

There is no chance of cure after relapse following initial
treatment. A routine policy of close hospital follow-up is
therefore not essential although it may contribute to symptom control for some patients.

## Practice points

1 Lumbar puncture carries a significant risk in patients
  with any chance of raised intracranial pressure. It is
  particularly hazardous in the presence of headache,
  nausea, lethargy, papilloedema and posterior fossa or
  temporal lobe tumours. The risk can be lessened by the
  use of a small calibre needle, and by very slow withdrawal of a very small amount of CSF. No more CSF
  should be withdrawn if the pressure is raised above
  150 mm of fluid.
2 Patients should be warned not to drive. If there has
  been no history of fitting, a driving licence may be
  applied for in the United Kingdom one year post-
  craniotomy. If there has been a history of fitting, a
  driving licence may be applied for if at least two years
  has passed since both the craniotomy and the last fit,
  whether or not the patient is on anticonvulsants.

3 Ataxia, nystagmus and diplopia may be due to phenytoin or carbamazepine toxicity: serum levels should be
checked.

4 It is not always kind to try to improve the neurological
status of terminally ill patients with high dose steroids:
sometimes this may increase awareness of their pre-
dicament.

## NOTES

# CHAPTER 18

# Breast Carcinoma

The incidence of breast carcinoma is approximately 85 per 100,000 women annually. About one in fifteen women, therefore, develops breast cancer and many of these patients will live for several years with disease which eventually proves fatal. The combination of high incidence and a disease course of relatively long duration results in breast cancer patients forming a large percentage of the workload of most doctors practising in oncology; thus this is a relatively long chapter.

Almost all malignant breast growths are adenocarcinomas, usually arising from the mammary ducts, but sometimes from the lobules. Non-invasive in-situ carcinoma is probably more common than invasive carcinoma, but it is not usually clinically apparent. It is not known what percentage of in-situ carcinomas become invasive but 50 per cent is a reasonable estimate. It is also reasonably certain that many carcinomas become invasive at a very early stage in their development.

There is a tendency for breast neoplasia to be multifocal, particularly in-situ lesions. For lobular carcinoma in-situ there is a high chance of involvement of the contralateral breast. Overall, approximately 10 per cent of women at some stage develop overt contralateral invasive carcinomas and this figure would be substantially higher if they survived longer after their first cancer.

Breast carcinomas have a great propensity to establish distant metastases at a very early stage in their development and as a result probably not more than 20 per cent of patients are at present curable. However, this disease can have an extremely long natural history and metastatic disease occasionally becomes apparent for the first time after ten to twenty years or even longer. The overall relative survival at five years is approximately 60 per cent.

The prognosis is worse for those with large primary

tumours and nodal involvement, and those with tumours showing a lack of differentiation or evidence of blood vessel or lymphatic invasion. It is also worse for patients with tumours lacking oestrogen and/or progestogen cell surface receptors, those showing amplification of certain oncogenes, and inflammatory carcinomas. Inflammatory carcinomas are usually rapidly growing diffuse growths which are characterised by a pronounced warmth and overlying erythema.

Two randomised studies of screening have demonstrated a reduction in breast cancer mortality by approximately 30 per cent in women aged 50–65 who received mammography. However, other studies have suggested that benefit of this order of magnitude is difficult to reproduce, and there is as yet no evidence that screening reduces overall mortality. No significant benefit has been described from screening in women under 50 years or from programmes involving the teaching and encouragement of breast self-palpation.

### Risk factors

Benign breast disease; family history; nulliparity; late first pregnancy; early menarche; late menopause; primary biliary cirrhosis; radiation; possibly dietary fat and alcohol.

### Spread

Lymphatic spread is very common and occurs via dermal lymphatics to neighbouring skin and sub-cutaneous tissues, and to axillary, supraclavicular, subclavicular, ipselateral internal mammary, mediastinal and hilar lymph nodes. Spread may occur from the latter to the adjacent lung and pleura; metastatic pleural effusions more commonly occur on the side of the involved breast.

Haematogenous spread is also extremely common, especially to bones, where the centripetal skeletal involvement is highly suggestive of dissemination via Batson's paravertebral venous plexus (to vertebrae, ribs, pelvis, proximal humeri and femora, and skull). Blood-borne spread also commonly occurs to lungs, liver and, to a somewhat lesser extent, bone marrow and brain.

## Symptoms and signs

Visible or palpable tumour
Breast pain (may indicate carcinoma even when no
tumour palpable)
Nipple retraction
Peau d'orange
Warmth/erythema
Nipple discharge/bleeding
Skin involvement/ulceration, including
Eczematous change around nipple (Paget's disease)
Deep fixation
Axillary/supra- and infra-clavicular lymphadenopathy
Bone pain
Dyspnoea/cough
Pleural effusion
Hepatomegaly
Ascites

# Treatment

### Radical

Surgery

Surgery remains the most effective treatment for operable
primary tumour and axillary lymphadenopathy. In many
patients smaller (<5 cm) localised tumours are easily macroscopically removed by local excision, wedge excision or quad-
rantectomy, but the chance of recurrence within the remaining breast is approximately 30 per cent following such
surgery alone. The chance of local recurrence following total
mastectomy is overall substantially less, but may approach
this level in some patients with larger tumours, tethering to
skin or chest wall and axillary lymphadenopathy. In both
instances the chance of loco-regional recurrence can be reduced by post-operative radiotherapy to 5–10 per cent.

There is little place now for the traditional radical mastectomy involving removal of the entire breast and skin over-

lying the tumour, pectoralis minor and major muscles and all the fibroareolar lymph node containing axillary tissue. This is because it confers no survival advantage compared with lesser procedures, and loco-regional control of disease is no better than with lesser surgery and radiotherapy.

Late reconstructions (at least 4–6 months after primary surgery) may be performed on some patients treated by mastectomy and can offer a substantial improvement in body image. Where there is some laxity in the skin over the anterior chest a silastic gel prosthesis may be simply implanted and closure achieved easily. Where the skin is tight, or where it has been damaged by radiotherapy, it is necessary to advance a flap of skin and underlying tissues to replace the defect. A latissimus dorsi myocutaneous flap is commonly used to cover an underlying prosthesis. There are techniques available to reconstruct a nipple and areola, but many women are satisfied with the basic reconstruction.

Loco-regional tumour control is important regardless of survival, because of the potentially appalling impact of uncontrolled disease on the chest wall or in lymph nodes on the quality of life. Mobile metastatic axillary lymphadenopathy is most effectively treated by surgery. Axillary exploration and node sampling can also be very helpful when there is no palpable lymphadenopathy because involved nodes are frequently impalpable, and because the finding of axillary nodal involvement gives prognostic information which may alter subsequent management, particularly in pre-menopausal women. (See section on cytotoxic chemotherapy.) A thorough axillary dissection up to the axillary vein remains a popular and effective method of preventing axillary relapse, although microscopic nodal involvement is as effectively dealt with by radiotherapy. An axillary dissection should not be followed by radiotherapy because the risk of lymphoedema (which can occur from either treatment when given alone) is very substantially increased. (See Chapter 8 Part I and sections on lymphoedema and mastectomy in Chapter 15.)

## Radiotherapy

This is usually given as an adjuvant to surgery. It is highly effective, when given post-operatively, in eliminating microscopic residual disease in the breast, chest wall or regional lymph nodes, but it has not been demonstrated to improve survival, although its use is increasing with the lesser use of mastectomy. It is not inconceivable that the improved local control achieved with radiotherapy following breast-conserving surgery may increase the chance of cure for the small minority of patients who have not developed viable micrometastases at the time of presentation. These patients will usually have very small tumours.

There are, however, substantial disadvantages from radiotherapy. It usually lasts four weeks or more, and inevitably causes marked skin soreness and sometimes severe moist desquamation, particularly underneath the breast and in the axilla. Skin telangiectasia occurs frequently in the long term, particularly at the site of a 'boost' dose (see below). Shoulder stiffness is also common after axillary radiation, and a small minority experience a frozen shoulder. Some pulmonary fibrosis is almost inevitable with external radiotherapy, but this is usually not symptomatic unless a substantial amount of lung is irradiated, or if there was previously impaired lung function. More serious still is the risk of cardiac damage following treatment of left-sided tumours, and the induction of second malignancies. A small increased risk of death arising from both these complications has been documented in patients given older techniques of radiotherapy but these risks may still apply to modern megavoltage methods. They may be particularly important in considering optimal treatment for patients with a good prognosis.

Most breast radiotherapy is given using external megavoltage beams which may or may not encompass regional lymph nodes as well as the breast or chest wall. A 'boost' dose is often given to the tumour bed after breast-sparing surgery because of the higher risk of recurrence at or near the original tumour site. This may be given using external beams of electrons or X-rays, but is also quite often given using interstitial techniques, often with radioactive iridium wires inserted into hollow plastic tubes threaded through the breast tissue. However this does not now seem to produce the better cosmetic result (compared with an external beam boost) that was once thought.

## Endocrine manipulation

This has no curative potential for clinically detectable tumour, but when given adjuvantly to local treatment it can improve the chance of medium-term (5–10 years) survival for some women. It is not yet known whether it can contribute to the chance of ultimate cure. The evidence for efficacy is best for the anti-oestrogen tamoxifen when given to post-menopausal patients for at least two years, usually in a dosage of 20 mg daily, although approximately 20 patients need to be treated in order to result in one extra survivor at five years. This treatment is usually very well tolerated and a large number of women benefit because this is such a common tumour. It is not yet known whether treatment beyond two years confers additional benefit. There is a low risk of retinopathy and other possible side effects from long-term tamoxifen but there is some evidence to suggest that it reduces the incidence of clinically apparent cancer in the opposite breast.

The evidence for benefit from adjuvant tamoxifen is somewhat less strong for pre-menopausal women, although two large British studies have shown benefit to be independent of menopausal status. There is also evidence of a survival benefit from adjuvant castration (oophorectomy or low dose radiation menopause) for pre-menopausal women, but again this is not as clear-cut as that for tamoxifen for post-menopausal patients (or adjuvant cytotoxic chemotherapy for premenopausal women). Trials are now in progress examining the efficacy of an adjuvant 'medical castration' using LH-RH agonist drugs.

## Cytotoxic chemotherapy

This also has no curative potential for clinically detectable tumour, but it has been shown to be effective as an adjuvant treatment in prolonging the survival of pre-menopausal patients, particularly those with metastatic axillary lymphadenopathy. Optimal chemotherapy for these patients is almost certainly combination chemotherapy, and the best tried regimen is a combination of cyclophosphamide, methotrexate and 5-fluorouracil (CMF) given for six months. It is again far too soon to draw conclusions about the ability of cytotoxic chemotherapy to contribute to cure, but the survival advantage has been shown to persist well beyond 10 years, with little sign of diminution. Nevertheless about 10 patients need to be treated for one extra survivor at five years. The percentage increase in survival seems comparable in both node positive and node negative patients, but the absolute improvement in the chance of survival is substantially greater in node positive patients. For these patients adjuvant cytotoxic chemotherapy is now considered standard treatment in the USA and its use is growing in Britain.

This is quite toxic treatment, both physically and psychologically. Nausea and vomiting and alopecia are common, but more distressing for many patients is the psychological trauma of treatment. It increases the incidence of clinically detectable anxiety and depression, which affects about one third of breast cancer patients following initial diagnosis and treatment. The psychological morbidity of chemotherapy may be particularly troublesome because no benefit can actually be seen by the patient; it seems to be substantially greater than that arising from treatment for overt disease where patients often experience an improvement in symptoms or may notice lumps getting smaller as a result of treatment.

There is controversy about the contribution of chemotherapy-mediated ovarian suppression to treatment efficacy. A substantial percentage of treated women stop having periods, but there is disagreement about whether or not these women derive greater benefit from treatment than those who continue to menstruate. For post-menopausal women the benefit from cytotoxic chemotherapy is rather less and the toxicity rather more. As a result tamoxifen appears to be a preferable option, although there is persisting enthusiasm for examining the rôle of adjuvant cytotoxic chemotherapy in post-menopausal women with a particularly poor prognosis.

## Palliative

### Surgery

For some patients surgery has a useful rôle to play in controlling loco-regional disease even when there can be little prospect of cure. This may involve excision of 'recurrences' in the breast or chest wall, 'toilet mastectomy' or excision of axillary lymphadenopathy. More extensive 'recurrent' disease on the chest wall may be usefully treated by wide excision and repair using flap rotation, and omental transposition has been very successful in some patients in providing a useful base for split-skin grafting, and in helping to 'police' local neoplasia. Surgery has little use in the management of distant metastases other than internal fixation for impending or established pathological fracture and decompressive laminectomy for spinal cord or cauda equina compression.

## Radiotherapy

This has an important place in the control of inoperable loco-regional disease, whether this is 'recurrent' tumour after initial treatment or in patients presenting with very advanced fixed or ulcerating carcinomas, or inflammatory carcinomas. Inflammatory carcinomas are usually best treated with cytotoxic chemotherapy followed by radiotherapy: this affords the best chance of a modest (more than two years) survival and loco-regional control.

Radiotherapy is very frequently employed in the palliation of painful bone metastases when one high dose fraction is usually adequate. Radiotherapy also has an important part to play in the management of spinal cord or cauda equina tumour compression where decompressive surgery is not considered appropriate due to the extent of disease, duration of symptoms or general condition of the patient.

A 'radiation menopause' (see below) is usually an acceptable alternative to surgical oophorectomy whether used adjuvantly or as treatment for advanced disease. The ovaries are very radiosensitive and can be ablated by a low dose of pelvic irradiation with minimal bowel disturbance. The full response usually takes two to three months, however, and surgery may be preferred for more rapidly progressive disease.

## Endocrine manipulation

This may include tamoxifen, progestogens, aminoglutethimide with steroid replacement, oophorectomy or radiation menopause and LHRH agonists. Other less used options include oestrogens, androgens, adrenalectomy and hypophysectomy: the last two are now very rarely performed. In general, endocrine manipulations are well tolerated, particularly tamoxifen and progestogens.

In about one third of patients there is a response to one or other of these hormonal manipulations. In addition approximately another 20 per cent of patients will benefit from having their disease stabilised. The most popular are tamoxifen and progestogens, for reasons of lack of toxicity and simplicity. The progestogens confer an additional benefit to some patients by improving their general sense of well-being, appetite and weight. The mean duration of response from hormonal manoeuvres is about nine months but some patients derive benefit for a few years; responses are sometimes very slow, taking a few months to become apparent. Approximately one third of patients will respond to another hormonal manoeuvre following relapse after a response from the first. Withdrawal responses are also seen following an initial response to treatment. This occurs in 15–20 per cent of patients on tamoxifen, particularly those with 'soft tissue' disease. The chance of a response to an alternative manoeuvre following initial failure is usually no higher than 10 per cent. Occasional responses are seen as a result of increasing tamoxifen in relapsing or non-responding patients from a standard dose of 20–40 mg/day to 100 mg/day. The addition of prednisolone 10 mg daily to tamoxifen or ovarian ablation has been shown to increase the response rate to almost 50 per cent and the mean duration of response by about four months.

Response rates to endocrine manoeuvres are highest in patients with well-differentiated tumours, relatively indolent disease, 'recurrence' which becomes manifest several years after primary treatment, older patients, those with 'soft tissue' disease (breast, lymph nodes, skin and subcutaneous tissue) and bone metastases, and those with tumours showing a high oestrogen and/or progestogen receptor content. Response rates are low for rapidly progressive and poorly differentiated carcinomas, particularly those involving lungs or liver.

## Cytotoxic chemotherapy

Several drugs, including cyclophosphamide, methotrexate, 5-fluorouracil, mitoxantrone and mitomycin C, produce responses in one-quarter to one-third of patients when given singly. Response rates approaching 50 per cent are seen with adriamycin and epirubicin, and several combinations of drugs produce response rates of 60 per cent and even higher. In general, the higher response rates are achieved with treatment that is more toxic; it has not been established that the initial use of combinations is advantageous compared with the use of single drugs used sequentially – neither has it been established that there is benefit from prolonging effective chemotherapy beyond 4–6 courses.

Cytotoxic chemotherapy is considerably more toxic than endocrine manipulation and should be used cautiously. In general it is not appropriate for frail or elderly patients and others with 'poor performance status'. It is most commonly considered after hormonal manipulations have failed, but it is often the first treatment of choice for rapidly progressive disease, particularly when involving lung or liver. It is also usually the preferred initial treatment for patients presenting with inflammatory carcinomas.

It can sometimes take a couple of months for a response to treatment to become apparent, but continued tumour growth at any time after the start of treatment indicates resistance. The mean duration of response from cytotoxic chemotherapy is usually 5–10 months. The response rates to 'second line' chemotherapy following an initial response are usually low, particularly if combination chemotherapy was used initially, and extremely low if there was no response initially; the chance of response does not, however, seem to be reduced by previous adjuvant chemotherapy. Survival is undoubtedly prolonged for some patients, but the impact of chemotherapy on survival overall appears to be minimal; for some non-responding patients it may well shorten survival as well as impair their quality of life.

## Combinations of systemic treatments

Higher response rates have been reported using combinations of hormonal manoeuvres and hormonal manoeuvres with cytotoxic chemotherapy. However there is no evidence that such combinations improve survival or quality of life compared with the sequential use of single modalities.

## Diphosphonates

The long-term oral administration of APD (see section on hypercalcaemia in Chapter 13 in Part I) in a dose of 300 mg daily has been shown to reduce the incidence of pathological fractures, severe bone pain and hypercalcaemia in patients with osteolytic metastases. This drug can cause nausea and vomiting, but is well tolerated by the majority of patients. Newer diphosphonates may offer the prospect of greater efficacy and lower toxicity.

## Follow-up

Prolonged hospital follow-up is appropriate for most patients since the majority will relapse at some stage, and effective treatment can usually be offered for palliation, sometimes over several years. Close follow-up is recommended for patients at a substantial risk of local relapse, for example those treated with breast-sparing surgery alone or those not given post-mastectomy radiotherapy for unfavourable tumours. Loco-regional recurrence is most effectively dealt with at an early stage: prompt control may exert a marked influence on quality of life and very occasionally may be curative.

## Practice points

1.  Negative mammography or fine-needle aspiration cytology does not exclude carcinoma: tissue should be obtained for histology if there is continuing clinical suspicion.
2.  Newly diagnosed patients should be screened for metastatic disease by a thorough history and examination, alkaline phosphatase and other liver enzyme estimations. This should ideally be completed prior to any definitive surgical procedure, and certainly prior to mastectomy. Isotope bone scans are not necessary in the absence of abnormal biochemistry or a history of bone pain.
3.  Where breast-sparing surgery is feasible there is evidence

that involving patients in the decision on the type of surgery to be undertaken reduces the incidence of subsequent anxiety and depression, at least in the short term. Psychological morbidity is made worse by adjuvant chemotherapy, but not by adjuvant radiotherapy.

4. Drain sites should be positioned with a thought to the possible requirement of their inclusion in a subsequent radiotherapy volume, i.e. preferably not far down the chest wall.

5. Following breast surgery active shoulder exercises should start immediately after leaving hospital in order to prevent troublesome stiffness (which incidentally may adversely affect correct positioning for radiotherapy). They should also be encouraged after axillary radiotherapy.

6. Lymphoedematous arms are at risk of severe cellulitis following minor trauma. Patients should wear long gloves when gardening or undertaking other similar risky activity, and any infection should be promptly treated with antibiotics (see section on lymphoedema in chapter on rehabilitation).

7. There is no benefit from giving a 'loading dose' of tamoxifen and 20 mg daily has been proved to be as effective as 40 mg daily in post-menopausal women.

8. Rash and drowsiness are quite common side effects after starting aminoglutethimide, but usually subside if it is continued. Cortisone (25 mg bd) or hydrocortisone (20 mg bd) steroid replacement must be given concurrently with aminoglutethimide in standard dosage ($\geqslant$250 mg bd).

## NOTES

# NOTES

# CHAPTER 19

# Bronchial Carcinoma

The incidence is approximately 70 per 100,000 population annually and the male/female ratio 3:1. Approximately 50 per cent are squamous carcinomas, 20 per cent small cell (oat cell) carcinomas, 20 per cent large cell carcinomas and 10 per cent adenocarcinomas. Tumours arise from a major bronchus in 75 per cent of cases, and a peripheral bronchus in 25 per cent. Mediastinal and supraclavicular fossa involvement may lead to superior vena caval compression, and to compression or invasion of phrenic, recurrent laryngeal and cervical sympathetic nerves.

A small number of squamous and adeno-carcinomas have an extremely long doubling time, show little change in size on sequential annual chest radiography and are compatible with survival for several years despite no treatment. The opposite extreme is far more common, however, and small cell carcinomas, in particular, tend to have short doubling times, the average being approximately only 30 days. Distant spread tends to occur early in lung cancer, particularly with small cell carcinomas where occult or overt spread has occurred in the great majority of patients by the time of diagnosis.

The overall five-year survival is approximately 7 per cent. Of the 20 per cent who have a 'curative' resection approximately one third will be alive at five years. The chance of cure is highest for patients with squamous carcinoma, and very low indeed for those with small cell carcinoma.

### Risk factors

Smoking (not adenocarcinomas); urban dwelling; asbestos; uranium and other metallic occupational exposures.

Spread

Direct spread occurs to the adjacent parenchymal lung tissue, mediastinum, pleura, chest wall, brachial plexus, diaphragm and pericardium, and submucosally up and down the bronchus. Lymphatic spread is very common and occurs principally to the hilar nodes, mediastinum and supraclavicular fossae. Haematogenous spread is also very common, and occurs especially to bones, liver and brain.

## Symptoms and signs

Cough
Haemoptysis
Dyspnoea
Chest pain
Wheeze/stridor
Pain in shoulder or down arm
Personality change or other evidence of brain metastases
Bone pain
Hepatomegaly
Supraclavicular lymphadenopathy
Superior vena caval obstruction
Hoarse voice from recurrent laryngeal nerve palsy
Horner's syndrome
Spinal cord or cauda equina compression
Paraneoplastic (non-metastatic) phenomena, eg
    weight loss
    clubbing
    gynaecomastia
    anaemia
    hypercalcaemia
    hyponatraemia due to inappropriate ADH secretion
    hypokalaemia and hyperglycaemia due to 'ectopic' ACTH
    neuromyopathies

# Treatment

## Radical

### Surgery

This is the best hope of cure. Contra-indications include superior vena caval obstruction, cytologically positive pleural effusion, extension to within 2 cm of the carina, nerve palsies, significantly impaired cardiac or lung function, and advanced biological age. Weight loss is also an ominous sign, strongly suggesting incurability. Approximately 30 per cent of patients will be thought suitable for radical surgery with either lobectomy or pneumonectomy. Surgery should be preceded by thorough staging investigations, including CT scanning and/or mediastinoscopy, performed in the attempt to exclude extensive regional or extrathoracic metastases. Approximately one third of these (10 per cent of the total) will be found to have inoperable disease at surgery. Pancoast tumours should not necessarily be considered inoperable: radical resection of localised tumours can occasionally be curative.

The mortality of pneumonectomy can be as high as 10 per cent, approximately three times as great as lobectomy. It also carries a greater risk of long-term cardiopulmonary morbidity. Thus lobectomy is preferable when a tumour is confined to one lobe and there is no lymphadenopathy. Approximately another 10 per cent of patients will experience severe postoperative morbidity, usually those undergoing pneumonectomy and older patients. Complications include cardiac dysrhythmia, haemorrhage, bronchopleural fistula, empyema and atelectasis of the remaining lung. Longer-term complications include severe respiratory insufficiency, cor pulmonale, and post-thoracotomy chest wall pain.

### Radiotherapy

Many of the contra-indications to surgery are also contra-indications to radical radiotherapy. However, carefully selected patients who decline surgery or who are considered medically unfit for it are suitable for radical radiotherapy, although the chance of cure is significantly less than with surgery. There is however some early evidence suggesting that accelerated hyperfractionated radiotherapy may be rather more effective than conventional regimens. Dysphagia due to radiation oesophagitis is almost inevitable. Radiation pneumonitis and subsequent fibrosis in the surrounding normal lung is inevitable, and may cause cough and dyspnoea 1–3 months after the completion of treatment, particularly if a large volume is treated. Symptomatic improvement may be achieved with steroids.

## Cytotoxic chemotherapy

This is curative for a very small percentage of patients with small cell carcinoma apparently confined to the chest. (See palliative section.)

## Combined modality

Various combinations of surgery, radiotherapy and cytotoxic chemotherapy have been tried and are under continued evaluation, but none has been proved to improve the chance of cure. However it is common practice to consider post-operative radical radiotherapy for some patients thought to have residual non-bulky intrathoracic tumour after surgery, and there is quite good evidence that the resectability of localised Pancoast tumours can be increased by pre-operative radiotherapy.

## Palliative

### Surgery

Bronchoscopic laser destruction of exophytic tumour is an effective palliative treatment, particularly for relatively central growths. Relief of airway obstruction leads to improvement in breathlessness, and haemoptysis is also relieved in the majority of cases. Treatment is carried out under general anaesthesia, is well tolerated and quick, but the duration of symptom relief is usually not more than three or four months. Photoradiation therapy is a type of laser treatment in which patients are injected with haematoporphyrin derivative (HPD) three days before the tumour is made the target of an argon dye laser. HPD is concentrated within tumour tissue and can be activated when the laser light is at the right frequency, resulting in local tissue destruction.

Oesophageal intubation is useful in patients with dysphagia due to compression by mediastinal glands, and in patients with an oesophago-respiratory fistula.

## Radiotherapy

Although it has little effect on the duration of survival, external radiotherapy remains the mainstay of palliative treatment. It is effective in relieving haemoptysis in over 80 per cent of patients, and over 50 per cent will experience improvement in breathlessness, cough, superior vena caval obstruction and pain in the chest, shoulder or arm. It is relatively ineffective for pleural effusion, and relief of recurrent laryngeal or phrenic nerve palsies is unusual. It is usually well tolerated but mild radiation oesophagitis is common. This usually comes on a week or two after the start of treatment, but rarely lasts for more than a few days unless high doses are used. High dose rate bronchoscopically guided intracavitary radiotherapy is now feasible and appears to offer comparable efficacy to external treatment whilst being completed much more quickly.

Metastases are very common in this disease and external radiotherapy is often required, and very effective, for painful bone lesions. For spinal cord compression radiotherapy is often preferred to surgical decompression because of the poor prognosis of these patients. Symptomatic relief from brain metastases is achieved in the majority of patients, particularly those with small cell carcinoma, which tends to be more radiosensitive than the other tumours, but alopecia is inevitable and dexamethasone is often the preferred initial option.

Prophylactic cranial irradiation is a component of some protocols of treatment incorporating cytotoxic chemotherapy for patients with apparently localised small cell carcinoma. It has no significant effect on survival but it does reduce the incidence of brain metastases. This can make terminal care easier and reduce the requirement for hospitalisation. Some small cell carcinoma protocols have also included chest irradiation in addition to cytotoxic chemotherapy. Overall this does not seem to have made much impact on survival, but it may slightly increase the low chance of long-term survival or cure.

## Cytotoxic chemotherapy

For patients with other than small cell lung carcinoma the response rates are relatively low, and there is no evidence that patients do better than if treated with palliative radiotherapy as necessary. Small cell carcinoma is much more responsive, particularly to combinations of three or four drugs (principally cyclophosphamide, adriamycin, vincristine and etoposide) and chemotherapy should be considered for most patients with these tumours. For patients with no overt evidence of distant spread, the median survival of about six months can be doubled with combination chemotherapy, and approximately 20 per cent are alive and well two years after diagnosis. A small number of patients ($\leqslant 5$ per cent) are alive and well after five years, and are probably cured. The response to chemotherapy is less satisfactory for those patients presenting with distant metastases but nevertheless for many this may still represent the best approach to palliation. Their median survival is prolonged from a few weeks to approximately 6–8 months. Regardless of whether or not there is overt metastatic disease, patients who have experienced significant weight loss or who have a poor 'performance status' tend to do very badly.

## Follow-up

There is virtually no chance of successful salvage after attempted curative treatment, and there is therefore no strong justification for routine clinical or radiological hospital follow-up. The patient and his own doctor should however be made aware of the possibility of (further) effective palliative treatment.

## Practice points

1.  Overt distant metastatic disease must be excluded prior to radical treatment with surgery or radiotherapy by a thorough clinical assessment and, at the least, by serum biochemistry including alkaline phosphatase and other liver enzyme estimations. Further investigations may be required, including an isotope bone scan and ultrasound or CT liver scan.

2.  Bronchial carcinoma is by far the commonest cause of paraneoplastic syndromes. These occur especially with small cell carcinoma but non-metastatic hypercalcaemia characteristically occurs with squamous carcinoma. Vigorous correction of metabolic abnormalities is often not kind.

3.  There is usually little point in telling longstanding smokers treated palliatively to give up smoking.

## NOTES

# CHAPTER 20

# Cervical Carcinoma

The incidence of invasive tumours is approximately 15 per 100,000 women annually. About 90 per cent are squamous carcinomas, and most of the remainder are adenocarcinomas, which arise either from the endocervical mucosa or mucus-secreting endocervical glands. The majority of invasive carcinomas are preceded by cervical intra-epithelial neoplasia (CIN, grades 1–3) and in most patients the duration of intra-epithelial neoplasia prior to the development of invasive carcinoma is probably ten years or more. Probably only about 10–15 per cent of cervical carcinomas become invasive very early on in their development and it seems likely that a substantial proportion of invasive carcinomas can be prevented by screening and the treatment of abnormal mucosa identified at colposcopy.

About 50 per cent of patients have Stage I tumours at diagnosis, 35 per cent Stage II, 10 per cent Stage III and 5 per cent Stage IV (see staging below). However, tumour volume, rather than tumour stage, is the single most important factor in predicting survival, although these are related. There is a great variation in tumour volume within any given stage. For Stage I tumours under 2 cm the five-year survival is approximately 90 per cent, but for those over 4 cm it falls to under 50 per cent; most survival figures are quoted according to stage. Overall the relative five-year survival rate is about 55 per cent: Stage I approximately 80 per cent, Stage II 55 per cent, Stage III 30 per cent and Stage IV 5 per cent. For women under the age of 40 with Stage I tumours the five-year survival falls to below 50 per cent: there is evidence that the disease in young women is becoming more aggressive with an increased incidence of nodal metastases. Recurrence after five years is most unusual.

### Risk factors

Age at first intercourse; multiple sexual partners; smoking; low social class: probably Human Papilloma Virus infection.

### Spread

Direct invasion is to the vagina, parametrium or uterine body. Lymphatic is more common than haematogenous spread, and takes place principally to pelvic nodes, then para-aortic nodes. Tumours confined to the cervix have about a 15 per cent incidence of pelvic nodal involvement but the incidence rises rapidly with increasing local spread. Approximately 50 per cent of patients with involved pelvic nodes have involved para-aortic nodes. Blood-borne distant metastases occur more commonly with more advanced tumours: in about 20 per cent of patients with Stage III tumours.

### Staging (invasive tumours)

I   Confined to uterus
    a  Micro-invasive – diagnosed only by microscopy
    b  More advanced

II  Beyond uterus but not to pelvic side wall or lower third vagina
    a  Without parametrial invasion
    b  With parametrial invasion

III Extension to pelvic wall, lower third vagina, or causing hydronephrosis or non-functioning kidney
    a  Involving lower third vagina, without pelvic wall extension
    b  Pelvic wall extension, hydronephrosis or non-functioning kidney

IV  Invasion of rectal or bladder mucosa or extension beyond true pelvis

## Symptoms and signs

Post-coital bleeding
Intermenstrual bleeding
Menorrhagia
Vaginal discharge
Frequency of micturition
Pelvic pain
Low back pain
Leg swelling
Supraclavicular lymphadenopathy

# Treatment

## Management of abnormal cervical cytology and CIN

Ideally all women with dyskaryotic or persistent inflammatory cells in their cervical smears should be referred for
colposcopy, regardless of the degree of abnormality. Mildly
dyskaryotic cells and persistent inflammatory changes are
both associated with an increased risk of CIN 3. Unfortunately the colposcopy service is often unable to cope with the
immediate referral of all women whose smears show mild
dyskaryosis. In this case such smears should be repeated at
3–6 months and patients referred if the abnormality persists.
If no abnormality is visible on colposcopy but cytology showed
CIN 2 or more abnormal change endocervical curettage
('shallow' or 'diagnostic' cone biopsy) should be performed.

Abnormal areas on colposcopy should be punch biopsied. If
histology shows CIN 1–3 and the full extent of the lesion is
visible, locally destructive treatment should be given with
cryosurgery or laser evaporation, or with diathermy under
general anaesthesia. These techniques have cure rates of
85–95 per cent after one treatment. Cytology should be
repeated at four-monthly intervals, with repeat colposcopy in
the event of persisting abnormality. If the full extent of the
lesion is not visible a shallow cone biopsy should be performed.

If evidence of micro-invasive carcinoma is present on histology from the punch biopsy, a diagnostic cone biopsy should be performed. If the lesion is very small and only minimally penetrating the stroma, the excision margin clear and there is no lymphatic or blood vessel invasion, a full therapeutic cone biopsy may be considered adequate treatment, particularly for young women who wish to retain their childbearing potential. For any more extensive invasive lesion a more radical approach is essential.

# Treatment of Invasive Cancer

## Radical

### Surgery

For most patients with Stage I tumours and for some selected patients with Stage IIa tumours both surgery and radiotherapy are acceptable options. Local practice varies according to tradition and expertise. Both interfere with sexual function, but in different ways, and in general there is a preference for surgery in younger women. Overall there does not seem to be any difference in the chance of cure.

For selected patients with micro-invasive carcinoma a conservative abdominal hysterectomy without pelvic lymph node dissection is often considered adequate. For patients with more deeply invasive disease a more radical operation is necessary. In order to obtain adequate clearance around the primary growth the paracervical tissues are usually cut at the pelvic sidewall, and a pelvic lymphadenectomy is also performed. This operation is frequently referred to as a Wertheim's hysterectomy, although Wertheim himself removed only the pelvic lymph nodes if they were enlarged and suspicious for macroscopic involvement. The operative mortality is about 0.5 per cent.

Adverse effects of a radical hysterectomy include a shortened vagina, atonic bladder due to denervation, stress incontinence, and rarely ureteral fistulae. Significant sexual dysfunction from the shortened vagina is unusual. One advantage for surgery over radiotherapy in younger women is that the ovaries can be safely conserved.

Recurrent disease after radical radiotherapy carries a very poor prognosis, but about 25 per cent of carefully selected patients with small volume central pelvic recurrence may be salvaged by radical hysterectomy. Surgery is more difficult after radiotherapy and the risk of complications is significantly greater. For all other patients with technically operable (central) pelvic recurrence exenterative procedures offer the only (and slim) chance of successful salvage. These may be partial (conservation of bladder or rectum) or total.

## Radiotherapy

There are two main forms of radiotherapy for uterine malignancy, *intracavitary* and *external*.

Intracavitary radiotherapy makes use of the endometrial and vaginal cavities as containers for radioisotopes. The insertion of radioactive caesium (little radium is used nowadays) enables the delivery of a very high dose to the central pelvis, which is particularly useful in treating Stage I or II tumours. The inverse square law ensures that the intensity of dose falls off rapidly away from the uterus, nevertheless the anterior rectal wall, rectosigmoid junction and bladder base do receive high doses which can lead to significant morbidity. Insertions are made under general anaesthesia and the radioactive sources are left in-situ usually from 12 to 48 hours depending on their activity. Intracavitary radiotherapy is often fractionated, two or more insertions being given, often at weekly intervals, but there are considerable variations in the schedules used.

There is now an increasing use of remote afterloading. (See Chapter 6.) In some centres this is done using not radiocaesium but very high activity sources of radiocobalt. This enables the treatment time to be measured in minutes rather than hours or days, and the treatment is delivered entirely in the operating-room.

Intracavitary radiotherapy is sometimes used as the sole treatment for early tumours. It cannot deliver a cancerocidal dose to pelvic lymph nodes however, and it is usually given before or after whole pelvic external radiotherapy. The more advanced the disease the more prominent the rôle of external radiotherapy, and for advanced tumours external radiotherapy is often given alone

External radiotherapy can successfully salvage about 25 per cent of patients who develop a pelvic recurrence after radical hysterectomy. It is also occasionally given for disease in para-aortic lymph nodes but the value of this treatment is controversial because the radiosensitivity of small bowel significantly limits the dose that can be given. Patients with disease that has spread this far are likely to have even more distant metastases beyond the radiation field.

The short-term side effects of pelvic radiotherapy include nausea, vomiting, diarrhoea, proctitis, frequency, dysuria and abdominal pain. In the longer term functional ovarian ablation is inevitable. Vaginal dryness is also inevitable and vaginal adhesions and stenosis very common. Other long-term side effects include subdermal fibrosis over the anterior and posterior pelvis, pelvic fibrosis, proctitis (including haemorrhagic rectal telangiectasia), sigmoiditis, malabsorption, bladder telangiectasia and contracted bladder. Severe morbidity is uncommon, but major surgery is occasionally required for visceral damage, including stricture, fistula and perforation. Symptomatic relief from radiation proctitis is often achieved with steroid enemas. The risk of induction of second malignancies appears to be very low.

## Combined modality

In some centres pre-operative radiotherapy is given for early tumours but there is no good evidence of benefit and the complication rate is probably higher.

External pelvic radiotherapy is usually given after surgery if tumour was found to extend close to the margin of excision, or if histologically positive nodes are discovered.

Following encouraging response rates achieved with certain regimens of cytotoxic chemotherapy (e.g. bleomycin, ifosfamide and cis-platinum) given as palliative treatment for advanced disease there are randomised trials in progress investigating the efficacy of chemotherapy as an adjuvant treatment for patients with an unfavourable prognosis. There is not yet any evidence that this improves survival.

## Palliative

### Surgery

Nephrostomy or ureterostomy should be performed in the presence of obstructive renal failure caused by pelvic tumour in patients who are eligible for radiotherapy, and in whom there is thus a very reasonable expectation of relieving the obstruction. Drainage should be performed very promptly since the serum potassium concentration can rise precipitously. Such procedures can, however, be unkind in the presence of clearly incurable disease as all that is achieved may be the replacement of one mode of death by a more unpleasant one a short time later.

Arterial ligation or embolisation can successfully control severe haemorrhage.

### Radiotherapy

This can have a very useful rôle even when cure is clearly not feasible, as in the very elderly and where there are distant metastases. The scope for further treatment after previous radical radiotherapy is however very limited.

### Cytotoxic chemotherapy

Response rates of about 70 per cent have been reported with some combinations of relatively toxic chemotherapy, and this is a reasonable option for selected patients.

## Follow-up

Long-term follow-up is essential for those with CIN. Patients with normal smears after treatment have a risk of invasive carcinoma approximately three times greater than normal and for those with abnormal smears after treatment the risk is very substantially higher.

About 80 per cent of recurrences of invasive carcinoma occur within two years. Since salvage treatment is occasionally successful for recurrence of Stage I and II tumours, close follow-up is justifiable for these patients for the first 3–4 years. Vaginal vault or cervical cytology can pick up early recurrences that are not clinically obvious, but cytological interpretation is often difficult after radiotherapy. It is sometimes clinically difficult to distinguish recurrence from radiation fibrosis or vault necrosis.

## Practice points

1 Overt metastatic disease must be excluded prior to radical treatment. Supraclavicular fossae examination, chest radiography, blood urea, electrolytes and liver function tests are essential. Abdominal computed tomography or lymphangiography may give very valuable further information, particularly with larger primary tumours.

2 Staging prior to radical treatment should routinely incorporate examination under anaesthesia (including cystoscopy) and intravenous urography.

3 Pre-menopausal women with squamous carcinomas treated with radiotherapy or who have had ovaries removed should be given oestrogen replacement (combined oestrogen/progestogen contraceptive pill) in order to avoid or reduce accelerated bone resorption, loss of libido, reduction of vaginal lubrication and decreased vaginal sensation. The rôle of oestrogen replacement after treatment for adenocarcinomas, which may be hormone responsive, is controversial.

4 Sexually active women should be advised to resume intercourse as soon as possible after radiotherapy, to prevent adhesions. Lubricating jelly is usually necessary. Non-sexually active women may be advised to perform regular self-dilatation; keeping the vagina patent makes follow-up pelvic examination much easier.

# NOTES

# CHAPTER 21

# Colorectal Carcinoma

The incidence is approximately 45 per 100,000 population annually and the male/female ratio 1:1. The colon/rectum ratio is 3:2 but 70 per cent of tumours arise in the rectum or sigmoid colon. Virtually all are adenocarcinomas. Some carcinomas arise from previously benign polyps. Polyps under 1 cm in diameter have only a 1 per cent incidence of carcinoma within them, but one third of polyps larger than 2 cm will show evidence of malignant change. Patients with a long duration of symptoms appear to have a better prognosis, presumably because their tumours are less aggressive. Young patients tend to have more aggressive tumours.

Overall approximately 25 per cent of patients are cured, but when the lymph nodes are not involved and there is no evidence of distant metastases (Duke's stages A & B), the cure rate rises to approximately 70 per cent. For patients with nodal involvement but no evidence of distant metastases (Duke's stage C) the chance of cure is about 20 per cent.

## Risk factors

Ulcerative colitis; Crohn's disease; intestinal polyps; familial history; coeliac disease; a low-fibre diet is probably numerically of far greater significance, but this is not yet established beyond all doubt.

## Spread

Through the bowel wall, to regional lymph nodes (discovered in 40 per cent at surgery), and via the blood stream, especially to the liver (discovered in 15 per cent at surgery).

## Symptoms and signs

Bleeding
Abdominal pain
Constipation
Diarrhoea
Nausea and vomiting
Tenesmus
Weight loss
Weakness
Anaemia
Abdominal or rectal mass
Hepatomegaly
Supraclavicular lymphadenopathy

# Treatment

## Radical

### Surgery

Resection of the primary tumour with or without nearby lymph nodes offers virtually the only chance of cure. Resection of relatively localised metastatic liver disease may be justified as this can probably improve disease-free survival, and possibly even result in cure for a small minority.

There should be wide excision margins to reduce the chance of local recurrence. Anastomotic recurrences are nevertheless quite common, due either to incomplete resection of invasive carcinoma, implantation or pre-malignant change in the residual bowel mucosa. The presence of abnormal (sialo) mucin at the resection margins on special staining identifies patients at higher risk of local recurrence due to pre-malignant change.

Tumours of the lower third of the rectum are usually treated by abdomino-perineal resection with a colostomy. (See Chapters 8 and 15.) Higher tumours are usually treated by an anterior resection with re-establishment of bowel continuity. Lower rectal tumours are not easily amenable to anterior resection because of the need to have a good inferior as well as superior excision margin, thereby militating against the preservation of anal sphincter function. However, modern stapling techniques have enabled anterior resection for tumours which would have hitherto been treated by abdomino-perineal resection. This approach sometimes leads to an increased incidence of local recurrence, although adjuvant radiotherapy may well be able to cope with this.

Meticulous excision of the rectal mesentery has been shown to be capable of reducing the requirement of permanent colostomy for patients with rectal carcinoma to almost 10 per cent, and of keeping the rate of local recurrence below 5 per cent. For rectal carcinoma the surgical technique may possibly be the most important factor in determining the outcome for patients with potentially curable tumours.

Complications of surgery include anastomotic leaks, infections and urinary and sexual dysfunction. The latter are largely consequent on direct physical trauma, pelvic nerve damage or psychological sequelae (particularly common with abdomino-pelvic resection). Between 25 per cent and 75 per cent of men report disturbances in sexual desire, erection or ejaculation after colorectal surgery. The overall mortality rate from surgery is approximately 5 per cent, although it is much higher in elderly patients.

## Radiotherapy

Abdominal radiotherapy is poorly tolerated and radiotherapy has almost no rôle in the radical treatment of colonic carcinoma. Pelvic radiotherapy is much better tolerated because of the presence of less small bowel, although all patients will experience intestinal side-effects to a greater or lesser extent. Conventional external beam therapy occasionally provides a cure for patients whose rectal tumours are considered inoperable or who are otherwise unfit for surgery.

In a few centres, notably in France and the USA, low-voltage radiotherapy is given for very superficial rectal tumours that can be reached by an applicator, inserted through the anus. Tumours suitable for this treatment probably constitute about 10 per cent of the total number of rectal carcinomas. The treatment is well tolerated and the results comparable with the best reported for surgery.

## Combined modality

Pre- or post-operative pelvic radiotherapy can reduce the incidence of pelvic recurrence of rectal carcinoma, with an improvement in disease-free survival, but there does not appear to be any significant improvement in actual survival. There is now some evidence that adjuvant treatment which includes 5-fluorouracil containing chemotherapy can improve five-year survival in patients with more advanced tumours, but the improvement is probably only of the order of 5 per cent or less, and seems to be confined to patients with rectal carcinomas. Such treatment can be rather toxic and at present there seems to be little justification for considering it as part of routine management.

## Palliative

### Surgery

Resection is justified for the relief of symptoms in those with inoperable metastases. A palliative defunctioning colostomy will relieve obstruction but it will not improve pain, bleeding, mucous discharge or secondary infection. It is quite often considered advisable prior to radical surgery or palliative radiotherapy for advanced tumours. Diathermy or cryosurgery may be used effectively to debulk exophytic rectal tumours, with relief of obstruction and an improvement in discharge and haemorrhage.

Liver metastases derive their blood supply predominantly from the hepatic artery and not the portal vein. Hepatic artery embolisation causes infarction in metastases and is frequently effective in the relief of pain, although it often causes a day or two of pain itself together with pyrexia. It is more effective than hepatic artery ligation as the subsequent development of a collateral circulation to the metastases is less likely.

### Radiotherapy

Palliative pelvic radiotherapy for inoperable or recurrent rectal carcinoma is usually relatively well tolerated. It is very effective in the relief of pain and bleeding and can also improve discharge. The duration of benefit is quite often one year or more. Hepatic irradiation is sometimes effective in the relief of pain from metastases, although upper abdominal radiotherapy often causes troublesome nausea and vomiting.

## Cytotoxic chemotherapy

Response rates are low, approximately 20 per cent, and the duration of response is usually only 3–6 months. However, one of the most effective drugs, 5-fluorouracil, is mostly well tolerated when given as a single agent. It is usually given intravenously. It can be given orally but its absorption is unpredictable. Higher response rates have been achieved with the concurrent administration of folinic acid, but this increases oral and gastro-intestinal toxicity. Higher response rates have also been reported using hepatic artery infusion, but this technique too has its complications and has not been shown to improve survival.

## Follow up

Patients who have had one colorectal carcinoma have an approximately 5 per cent chance of developing another. This risk is considerably increased if they have adenomatous polyps in addition to their cancer. They are of course at a greater risk of developing a recurrence of their first growth. The possibility that further surgery might lead to successful removal of an 'early' recurrence has led to some enthusiasm for routine 'second look' operations. However, problems arise from operative morbidity and mortality in patients who are not found to have recurrent tumour and there appears to be little justification for adopting 'second look' surgery as a routine procedure without any other evidence of recurrence.

Carcino-embryonic antigen (CEA) is a potentially sensitive tumour marker which may be used to detect a recurrence before it is detectable clinically or by other investigations. The serial serum measurement of CEA (e.g. 1–2 monthly for three years, then 3–4 monthly up to five years) has been extensively used in the follow-up of patients with colorectal carcinoma, as well as those with some other tumours. Approximately 75 per cent of colorectal carcinomas produce CEA. However, there are many non-neoplastic causes of a raised serum CEA concentration, including smoking, non-malignant hepatic, gastrointestinal, lung, renal and pancreatic disease, and a trend rather than a single elevated result should be the basis for considering a 'second look' operation. Although it has been reported that an increase in serum CEA occurs relatively late in patients with recurrent growth, approximately one third of those undergoing 'second look' surgery for a recurrence detected by serial CEA estimation will be cured.

It has been recommended that, in addition to serial CEA estimations, six monthly colonoscopies be performed for the first two years after primary surgery, principally with the aim of detecting a recurrence at the suture line, and that subsequently a barium enema or colonoscopy be performed every 2–3 years with the aim of detecting a second primary. This follow-up policy has not been subject to a randomised controlled trial, but it seems likely that it could save some lives, albeit at substantial cost.

## Practice points

1 Severe pelvic pain ± sciatica occurring within five years of surgery for rectal carcinoma is virtually diagnostic of recurrence in the absence of any other obvious cause. Usually there is no palpable abnormality and quite often a CT scan also fails to show tumour.

2 Some advanced apparently rectal tumours are in fact prostatic carcinomas. If the tumour is anterior, inseparable from the prostate or if there are urinary symptoms, immunohistochemistry for prostatic acid phosphatase or prostate-specific antigen should be performed. Diagnosis of a prostatic carcinoma has important implications for treatment in view of possible hormone-responsiveness.

# NOTES

# CHAPTER 22

# Endometrial Carcinoma

The incidence is approximately 13 per 100,000 women annually. The great majority of malignant tumours are adenocarcinomas and are clinically confined to the uterine body at presentation (Stage I). Most are well differentiated and relatively indolent tumours. A small number have squamous or sarcomatous components. Differentiation between well-differentiated carcinoma and endometrial hyperplasia can be difficult.

This disease tends to occur in an older age group than cervical carcinoma. Many patients are obese, and hypertension and diabetes are quite common. Obesity predisposes to this tumour due to the presence in adipose tissue of aromatase which converts endogenous adrenal androstenedione to oestrogen. Unopposed (without concomitant progestogen) oestrogenic stimulation causes both endometrial hyperplasia and carcinoma. Endometrial carcinoma cells often exhibit hormone receptors and almost half of these tumours are hormone-responsive.

The overall relative five-year survival is about 65 per cent: for Stage I tumours 75 per cent, but for Stage II tumours (cervical involvement) 50 per cent. For more advanced disease the five-year survival is ≤25 per cent. If there is no, or only superficial, myometrial invasion the five-year survival is over 80 per cent, but it falls to 50 per cent or lower where there is deep invasion. The prognosis is also influenced by the degree of differentiation and it is particularly poor when there is histological evidence of blood vessel invasion.

Risk factors

Obesity; nulliparity; unopposed oestrogen replacement; diabetes; hypertension.

Spread

Local spread occurs through the myometrium and inferiorly to the cervix. Lymphatic spread is to pelvic and para-aortic nodes and its incidence is considerably increased when there is deep invasion of the myometrium and in poorly differentiated tumours. Blood-borne spread is principally to lungs and liver.

## Symptoms and signs

Post-menopausal bleeding (90 per cent of patients are post-menopausal)
Vaginal discharge
Obesity
Hypertension (30 per cent)
Diabetes (20 per cent)

# Treatment

## Radical

Surgery

This offers the best chance of cure but, because of their age and frequent medical complications, the relatively low incidence of pelvic node involvement in Stage I patients and the lack of convincing evidence of benefit from lymphadenectomy, surgery for these patients is usually less radical than for those with cervical carcinoma.

Total abdominal hysterectomy and bilateral salpingo-oophorectomy is the treatment of choice for most patients although a more radical hysterectomy and lymphadenectomy is sometimes recommended for patients with Stage II tumours. A wide vaginal cuff is usually taken in order to reduce the risk of vault recurrence.

## Radiotherapy

Intracavitary radiotherapy has a lower potential for cure than surgery, but is the treatment of choice for those patients considered unfit for surgery.

## Combined modality

Pre-operative intracavitary radiotherapy has been widely practised, with the aim of reducing vault recurrence. However, the incidence of vault recurrence is dependent on surgical technique and is very low in some centres where pre-operative radiotherapy is not given. Most vault recurrences can be successfully treated by intracavitary radiotherapy and pre-operative treatment has not been shown to improve the chance of survival. External pelvic radiotherapy is often given after surgery when the tumour is found to be deeply invading the myometrium. Such treatment reduces the chance of pelvic recurrence but has not been shown to improve significantly the chance of survival. The side effects of radiotherapy are the same as for carcinoma of the cervix but they are more poorly tolerated in this population of older and generally less fit patients.

Almost half of endometrial carcinomas are hormone responsive. It has been claimed that the giving of progestogens at the time of initial treatment improves the chance of cure but the one randomised trial addressed to this concept has failed to substantiate this claim.

## Palliative

### Surgery

This has very little palliative use.

### Radiotherapy

This disease is not as radioresponsive as cervical carcinoma but radiotherapy can have a palliative rôle, principally in the control of bleeding.

## Cytotoxic chemotherapy

Response rates are low and it is virtually useless.

## Endocrine therapy

Progestogen treatment (medroxyprogesterone or megestrol) is always worth trying in advanced disease. The response rate overall is about 40 per cent with well-differentiated tumours being most likely to respond. Such treatment is usually very well tolerated and it should be continued for at least three months before concluding that it is not efficacious.

## Follow-up

Regular follow-up for five years is justified for most patients after potentially curative treatment, since recurrence in the vagina can be asymptomatic when still small, and can be successfully treated.

**NOTES**

# NOTES

# CHAPTER 23

# Head and Neck Carcinomas (Excluding Skin and Thyroid)

The total annual incidence is approximately ten per 100,000 population. The commonest single site of origin is the larynx (annual incidence approximately four per 100,000 population). In decreasing order of frequency other sites of origin are pharynx (naso-, oro- and hypo-), tongue, sinuses (maxillary antrum, ethmoid and sphenoid), salivary glands, lips, floor of mouth, nose and gums. The great majority of these carcinomas are squamous carcinomas, although adenocarcinomas constitute the majority arising from the salivary glands (major and minor), and a minority of tumours of the sinuses and nasal cavity, arising from mucus-secreting glands. For the squamous carcinomas there is a marked male preponderance, reflecting the aetiological importance of alcohol and tobacco.

As well as carcinomas, lymphomas arise in this region, particularly from Waldeyer's ring lymphoid tissue in the pharynx (including the tonsils). They are quite often truly localised to the head and neck, substantially more so than lymphomas presenting at other sites.

It is relatively unusual for any of the carcinomas to spread outside the head and neck region. Most treatment failure is due to a failure to achieve local control, and in this extremely cosmetically and functionally important part of the body this failure has devastating physical and psychological consequences. For some tumours surgical extirpation is not feasible because of local extent or site. For many others surgery is feasible but has a major impact on function and appearance. Radiotherapy is thus a very important modality for these tumours, and is the initial treatment of choice for the majority.

Overall almost 50 per cent of patients with these carcinomas are cured, but the prognosis varies greatly with the site and extent of disease. Tumours which tend to present at an early stage, e.g. carcinomas of the lip, anterior tongue and vocal cords are cured in the majority of cases, whilst the chance of cure for carcinomas of the oropharynx (including base of tongue), hypopharynx and supra- or infra-glottic larynx is only about 20–30 per cent. For each site there is marked variation according to the size of the tumour and whether or not there are involved lymph nodes. For small tumours confined to the vocal cord with no impairment of cord mobility or neck node involvement the cure rate is about 90 per cent; for large laryngeal tumours with extensive supra-glottic or sub-glottic involvement and involved neck nodes the chance of cure is less than 20 per cent. If lymph nodes are fixed the chance of cure is negligible, and the only realistic aim of treatment is palliation.

### Risk factors

Smoking and alcohol, particularly the combination; chronic irritation from ill-fitting dentures or repeated trauma; tobacco or moist snuff chewing; betel nut/slaked lime chewing; leucoplakia; Plummer-Vinson syndrome (oral cavity, oro- and hypo-pharynx); Epstein-Barr virus (nasopharynx); occupational exposure to wood dust and furniture manufacturing (adenocarcinomas of nasal cavity or sinuses).

### Spread

Local invasion and destruction can occur in any direction, including through bone, e.g. base of skull from nasopharynx. Lymphatic spread is extremely common, most commonly to submandibular or anterior neck triangle nodes, but nasopharyngeal carcinomas have a particular propensity to involve nodes in the posterior triangles, and bilaterally. Submental and pre-auricular nodes are not frequently involved. Perineural spread is quite common, and may cause pain. Blood-borne spread occurs principally to lungs and occasionally bones, but is much less frequent than lymphatic spread.

## Symptoms and signs

Hoarse voice
Ulceration
Pain
Impaired swallowing
Lymphadenopathy
Cranial nerve palsies (nasopharyngeal carcinoma)

# Treatment

## Radical

### Surgery

This is usually considered the primary treatment of choice for the relatively radioresistant adenocarcinomas. In some centres it is also preferred for some advanced squamous carcinomas and those invading the mandible, where the chance of success with radiotherapy is considered low. Where possible, involved lymph nodes are removed in continuity with the primary growth in an *en bloc* resection. Much surgery in this region is carried out as a potential salvage procedure following failure of radiotherapy. Radiation fibrosis can make surgery more difficult but only rarely renders it impossible.

The most frequent operation for primary tumours of the head and neck is laryngectomy. This is most commonly a total laryngectomy, although for a few tumours a supraglottic laryngectomy is feasible, leaving an airway and the vocal cords intact. For all others the creation of a tracheostomy is inevitable. Subsequent speech therapy is routine, but only about one-third of patients eventually manage good oesophageal speech. For others effective communication is feasible using a buzzing device (electrolarynx) applied to the floor of the mouth during normal articulation.

Surgery is usually considered the treatment of choice for patients who develop lymphadenopathy after successful treatment to a primary growth. This is partly because of the tendency for overt nodal disease to be relatively radioresistant, and partly because the tissue involved has often already been irradiated. A radical neck dissection is usually the preferred option because of the high likelihood of microscopic involvement of other nodes on the same side of the neck. This usually involves the removal of superficial and deep cervical fascia with contained anterior triangle nodes, sternomastoid muscle, internal and external jugular vein, accessory nerve and submandibular salivary gland, although more limited operations may sometimes be performed.

Major surgery in this region often requires substantial reconstruction using the patient's own tissues and/or prostheses. This may be performed at the time of removal of the tumour, or subsequently. Such surgery is frequently carried out by ENT surgeons and plastic surgeons working together.

## Radiotherapy

In many centres the routine treatment policy for most patients is initial radiotherapy followed by salvage surgery if necessary. Most radiotherapy is delivered by external megavoltage beams, but a small number of patients with small tumours at accessible sites, e.g. anterior tongue and lip, are suitable for brachytherapy using implants or surface applicators. External radiotherapy is sometimes recommended as an elective procedure following primary surgery. This is done when it is considered that there is a high likelihood of local recurrence, e.g. following surgery for malignant salivary gland tumours (and often following surgery for benign salivary pleomorphic adenomas), and also when there is doubt about the adequacy of resection for any other tumour. Preoperative radiotherapy is quite often recommended for tumours of the maxillary antrum. Radiotherapy is only very rarely successful when given for recurrence following primary surgery.

External radiotherapy to this region requires accurate planning and delivery. The treatment volume is often very close to crucial normal structures such as spinal cord, brain stem and eyes, which, whenever possible, need to be excluded from the high-dose region. In order to facilitate accuracy most patients will have a well-fitting mould made before the treatment is planned, and will have their treatment in it while it is fixed to the treatment couch. This ensures immobilisation, and the entrance and exit points of the beams are also marked on it. (See Chapter 6 in Part I.)

External radiotherapy is usually given over 3–6 weeks and can be extremely unpleasant, especially when large volumes are irradiated. Acute mucous membrane and skin reactions begin after about two weeks and often become severe. It is often advisable to admit these patients to hospital, particularly during the latter half of treatment and until the acute reaction shows some sign of subsiding. This is often not until a week or more after the completion of treatment.

Particular attention should be given to the maintenance of good hydration and adequate nutrition. Partial symptomatic relief can be achieved with topical agents such as local anaesthetics, aspirin gargles etc., and if necessary systemic analgesics and mild sedation may be given. Mucosal candidiasis is very common and requires prompt treatment with frequent (1–2 hourly) topical anti-fungal preparations. To the inexperienced eye, radiation mucositis can often look much like candidiasis: whenever there is doubt a swab should be taken.

Attention to the airway is very important in patients receiving treatment for bulky laryngeal tumours. Some patients may have slight inspiratory stridor at presentation, not severe enough to require a tracheostomy, but radiation oedema can substantially further compromise the airway. Dexamethasone is often useful but some patients do need a tracheostomy during the course of treatment.

Taste disturbance is almost universal when the mouth is irradiated and can persist for a very long time after treatment. Mouth dryness is also very common, particularly when both parotid glands are within the treatment volume. The qualitative and quantitative change in saliva predisposes strongly to caries and gum disease, and there is a consequent risk of osteitis of the jaw.

## Cytotoxic chemotherapy

This has been given prior to local treatment with radiotherapy or surgery, and synchronously with radiotherapy for patients with more extensive tumours. Although with some drugs and combinations squamous carcinomas show substantial regression in over half the patients, there is little evidence that this increases the chance of cure. What evidence there is is rather stronger for synchronous administration, but this increases the acute toxicity of radiotherapy, and the impact on the therapeutic ratio is uncertain. Drugs showing activity against squamous carcinomas in this region include methotrexate, 5-fluorouracil, bleomycin and the platinum compounds. The rôle of chemotherapy in radical treatment is under continuing evaluation in randomised trials.

## Palliative

### Surgery

Tracheostomy is the only commonly practised palliative surgical procedure in this region.

### Radiotherapy

Patients who have very extensive tumours, and the frail and elderly, may not be considered suitable for radical treatment because of the very low chance of cure and the inevitable toxicity. Nevertheless, many derive useful short-term benefit from intermediate dose radiotherapy. For some patients, however, the kindest option is just symptomatic medication.

### Cytotoxic chemotherapy

Fifty per cent or more of patients with advanced squamous carcinomas may be expected to show substantial tumour regression with some chemotherapeutic regimens, particularly patients with fairly rapidly growing exophytic tumours. Some combinations are fairly well tolerated and indeed may be less upsetting than radiotherapy. However, the efficacy of chemotherapy is much reduced in patients already treated with radiotherapy.

## Follow-up

Close follow-up is appropriate for all patients treated with curative intent, since early detection of relapse in either the primary site or neck nodes may lead to successful salvage. For squamous carcinomas 80 per cent of recurrences occur within the first two years. Most patients should be seen 1–2 monthly for the first year, 2–3 monthly for the second year and at greater intervals subsequently. The chance of recurrence after five years is extremely low.

## Practice points

1 It is important that all patients with residual teeth who are about to undergo irradiation to the region of the mouth have an expert dental assessment, and are given advice about long-term care to teeth and gums.
2 Tracheostomy patients must be educated on stoma care. Swimming should be avoided and bathing done with care. A protective bib should be worn when taking showers. The stoma should be covered with a thumb in order to develop an effective Valsalva manoeuvre during defaecation. Patients should be encouraged to wear medical alert bracelets, and to carry a card containing advice on pulmonary resuscitation technique.
3 Removal of the spinal accessory nerve in a neck dissection results in paralysis of trapezius, which can eventually lead to dropping of the shoulder, and pain. To prevent these late sequelae patients should be instructed in correct positioning of the arm, and in appropriate passive and active exercises.

# NOTES

# CHAPTER 24

# Hodgkin's Disease

This is less common than non-Hodgkin's lymphoma – approximately three new cases occur per 100,000 population annually. The male/female ratio is 3:2, and there is a bimodal age distribution with peaks in young adulthood and the elderly. Characteristically the malignant cell is the large 'Reed-Sternberg' cell containing two or more mirror image nuclei, each of which has a prominent large nucleolus. These cells are probably derived from the B-lymphocyte series. There is a large reactive cell population present within the tumour, comprising lymphocytes, plasma cells and fibrous tissue and in some patients the Reed-Sternberg cells are so few they can be very hard to find on histological examination. In some patients there is another type of malignant cell. These are uninucleate, found in 'lacunae' within the surrounding reactive cell population, and called Hodgkin's or lacunar cells. They do however retain the large nucleolus characteristic of the Reed-Sternberg cell.

There are four main types of Hodgkin's disease: lymphocyte predominant, nodular sclerosing, mixed cellularity and lymphocyte depleted, with a progressive increase in the proportion of Reed-Sternberg cells present and in the aggressive potential of the disease. In nodular sclerosing disease there is a very prominent fibrous tissue reactive component and the prognosis varies according to the cellular composition of the non-fibrous component – types I and II are recognised.

Lymphadenopathy is the principal feature of Hodgkin's disease. Unlike non-Hodgkin's lymphoma this disease tends to spread to contiguous lymph nodes and is far more often localised to one lymph node group or one part of the body. The lymph nodes involved tend to be those in the midline or major clinically accessible areas – involvement of sub-occipital or mesenteric nodes, for example, is unusual. Splenomegaly is quite common and may be due to actual involvement or a reactive change. Liver involvement also occurs in advanced disease but involvement of non-reticulo-endothelial tissues is unusual. In contrast to non-Hodgkin's lymphoma, marrow involvement is relatively uncommon (<5 per cent).

Involvement of nodes above the diaphragm, particularly in the neck, is more common than those below. Although the predominant route of spread is via lymphatics to contiguous nodes, splenic and liver involvement occur as a result of blood-borne spread. Hodgkin's disease is staged as follows: Stage 1 – involvement of a single lymph-node region or extralymphatic site (1E); Stage 2 – involvement of $\geq 2$ lymph-node regions or $\geq 1$ lymph-node region plus a single extralymphatic site on one side of the diaphragm (2E); Stage 3 – involvement of lymph-node regions on both sides of the diaphragm $\pm$ the spleen (3S) or another single extralymphatic site (3E); Stage 4 – diffuse or disseminated involvement of extralymphatic tissues, including liver or marrow. Each stage is subdivided into A or B according to the absence or presence of systemic symptoms respectively (see below).

Hodgkin's disease can be very indolent, with waxing and waning lymphadenopathy occurring over many months or even years. It can also be extremely aggressive – particularly the rare lymphocyte depleted variety. 'Recurrent' disease is sometimes of a more unfavourable histological type than at presentation. Overall about 75 per cent of patients are now cured. The cure rate is about 90 per cent for patients with localised non-bulky disease, favourable histology, a low ESR and no systemic 'B' symptoms (see below). The chance of cure falls to 50 per cent or lower for those with aggressive widespread disease and 'B' symptoms. Other adverse prognostic factors are male sex, increasing age, and bulky mediastinal disease.

### Risk factors

None is proven though there is epidemiological evidence implicating a common viral infection in the aetiology, possibly Epstein-Barr virus.

## Symptoms and signs

Painless rubbery lymphadenopathy
Splenomegaly
Night sweats ⎫
Weight loss >10 per cent ⎬ 'B' symptoms
Recurrent fever >38° ⎭
Pruritus
Tumour pain after ingestion of even very small amounts of alcohol.

---

# Treatment

---

### Radical

Surgery

This is largely limited to establishing the diagnosis or extent of the disease. Residual lymphadenopathy after radiotherapy or chemotherapy may be excised and sometimes is found not to contain any residual malignancy. Staging laparotomies are now relatively rarely performed. Normally, a staging laparotomy comprises inspection and palpation of all intra-abdominal and pelvic nodal groups, biopsies from a sample of nodes even if these appear normal, splenectomy, liver and iliac crest marrow biopsies. In younger women it may include oophoropexy (relocation of the ovaries) outside any proposed pelvic radiation field.

Staging laparotomy reveals infra-diaphragmatic disease that is not detectable by non-invasive methods in about 30 per cent of patients with disease otherwise apparently confined above the diaphragm. However, the increasing use of cytotoxic chemotherapy for patients with supradiaphragmatic disease with poor prognostic features, and the efficacy of chemotherapy as a salvage treatment for failure following local or regional radiotherapy above the diaphragm, have both been influential in the decreasing enthusiasm for staging laparotomy. It undoubtedly avoids unnecessary radiotherapy for some patients, but has its own hazards, and has not been shown to improve the chance of ultimate cure. Significant post-operative morbidity occurs in about 10 per cent of patients and there is a mortality risk of about 1 per cent. Splenectomy carries a long-term susceptibility to infection, especially with pneumococci and *Haemophilus influenzae*. Although this is particularly a problem in children, adults are also at risk. Infection in these patients can be dramatically sudden, overwhelming and fatal, especially pneumococcal septicaemia. Patients should receive polyvalent pneumococcal vaccine at least 2 weeks prior to splenectomy and oral long-term low dose penicillin prophylaxis subsequently (if not allergic).

## Radiotherapy

This disease is highly radiosensitive and is eradicated within the radiation volume in over 90 per cent of patients receiving intermediate dose radiotherapy, usually given over about four weeks. Nowadays radiotherapy is usually given only to patients with disease confined to one side of the diaphragm and no systemic symptoms (Stage I or IIA). 'Total nodal' irradiation ('mantle' plus 'inverted Y' fields [see below], separated by a month or so) is an effective treatment for Stage IIIA disease but is usually more upsetting than chemotherapy.

Radiotherapy may be localised merely to the involved nodes and a surrounding margin of about 5 cm, or is sometimes given to a larger volume in order to sterilise possible microscopic spread to contiguous nodes. Above the diaphragm such wide-field irradiation may take in the neck, supra- and infraclavicular fossae, axillae and mediastinum. The very radiosensitive lungs are substantially shielded and the irradiated volume is termed a 'mantle' field. Such treatment causes oesophagitis, sore skin and mouth, usually some occipital alopecia and some pneumonitis. However these side effects are rarely prolonged or unduly troublesome. Spinal cord irradiation may result occasionally in shooting pains down the legs on neck flexion (Lhermitte's sign) some months after treatment but this too is almost always self limiting. Permanent radiation myelopathy is very rare.

Treatment below the diaphragm, if extending to the pelvis (a treatment volume encompassing para-aortic and pelvic lymph nodes is termed an 'inverted Y' field), will inevitably cause infertility in females unless oophoropexy has been performed. There is also an appreciable risk of male infertility, although this can be reduced by testicular lead shielding. Wide-field infradiaphragmatic radiotherapy commonly causes nausea and vomiting. Diarrhoea is inevitable, although this is usually fairly well controlled and transient with the dose levels used.

The risk of relapse is generally lower with wide-field than more localised radiotherapy, but as salvage treatments enjoy a fairly high success rate it has not been shown to confer a survival advantage compared with localised treatment, and it carries greater morbidity.

## Cytotoxic chemotherapy

Combinations of drugs are essential for curative chemotherapy. A very well-known and established regimen is MOPP (mustine, oncovin [vincristine], procarbazine and prednisolone) given in monthly cycles. Usually at least 6–8 cycles are given, or at least three after the clinical disappearance of tumour. Other combinations are also used, some of which are rather less toxic and probably equally efficacious, e.g. LOPP in which leukeran (chlorambucil) is substituted for mustine.

Male sterility is common and usually irreversible. Female infertility is less common, particularly in younger women. A small percentage of patients will develop acute leukaemia or non-Hodgkin's lymphoma ten years or more after treatment; this is probably more common in those who have also received radiotherapy. It has been claimed that the risk of second malignancy is lower with an ABVD (adriamycin, bleomycin, vinblastine and DTIC) regimen. Higher response rates have been reported with alternating regimens, e.g. LOPP/EVAP (etoposide, vinblastine, adriamycin, prednisolone), but no survival benefit has yet been demonstrated.

## Combined modality

The use of combined chemotherapy and radiotherapy also leads to higher remission rates and improved disease-free survival, but again there has been little evidence of an actual survival advantage and the risk of induction of second malignancies is probably greater. However, many consider combined modality treatment to be necessary for patients with very bulky disease, particularly in the mediastinum.

## Bone marrow transplantation

Autologous bone marrow transplantation following very high dose chemotherapy is an experimental approach for some patients with relapsed disease and a very poor prognosis. It may be considered particularly justifiable for this chemo- and radio-responsive malignancy that relatively infrequently involves the bone marrow. About 10–20 per cent of patients refractory to conventional treatments may be expected to be alive and still in complete remission 2–3 years after autologous transplantation. This treatment has only been attempted relatively recently for patients with Hodgkin's disease, and there is as yet no evidence concerning its longer-term efficacy.

## **Palliative**

## Radiotherapy

Quite low dose radiotherapy can relieve symptoms from troublesome tumour masses in patients with widespread chemo-refractory tumour. Low dose irradiation can also relieve alcohol-induced tumour pain.

## Cytotoxic chemotherapy

This is usually given with curative intent but it may still provide useful palliation in patients whose disease has recurred after two or more attempts at cure, and for whom cure may seem extremely unlikely. Indeed it is important to recognise a 'chronic relapsing' type of Hodgkin's disease where cure is at present impossible but where symptomatic relief may be achieved with only one or two courses: more treatment is often unjustified, and can further compromise marrow reserve.

## Corticosteroids

These can improve the general sense of well-being, relieve B symptoms and sometimes slightly reduce tumour bulk.

## Follow-up

Prolonged hospital supervision is appropriate for most patients. Patients who relapse may be cured by further treatment with radiotherapy or chemotherapy.

## Practice points

1 Clinical staging normally involves estimation of the full blood count, plasma viscosity or ESR, serum biochemistry and chest X-ray, with CT scanning of chest and abdomen/pelvis for most patients. Bone marrow trephine and aspirate will indicate involvement in under 10 per cent of cases, usually only in patients with advanced disease, and they can be omitted in patients with localised good prognostic disease.

2 Clinical evidence of recurrence should be confirmed histologically, particularly in view of the long-term risk of non-Hodgkin's lymphoma.

3 Anti-pneumococcal vaccine should be given at least two weeks prior to splenectomy (although the antibody response is often impaired) and long-term low dose penicillin subsequently, as prophylaxis against pneumococcal septicaemia. The risk of this complication is particularly marked in children and adolescents. All splenectomised patients should be told that very prompt attention is required for any unexplained pyrexia.

4 Hodgkin's disease particularly suppresses T-cell immunity. Live vaccines are contra-indicated, probably for life.

5 Reactive splenomegaly and hepatitis are both quite common: mild splenic enlargement and raised liver enzymes do not necessarily indicate malignant involvement of these organs.

6 Small volume residual tumour after an otherwise

satisfactory response to treatment does not necessarily contain persistent malignant cells. Residual benign masses are particularly a feature of nodular sclerosing disease.

## NOTES

# CHAPTER 25

# Acute Leukaemias

The annual incidence is about four new cases per 100,000 population. These neoplasms arise from either lymphoid or myeloid stem cells. The malignant cells have a primitive, undifferentiated appearance and are known as *blast cells*. In children the majority of acute leukaemias are lymphoblastic (ALL), whilst in adults the majority are myeloid (AML). Both groups can be subdivided according to various morphological criteria and immune typing with monoclonal antibodies, and such classification has important implications for the response to treatment.

The leukaemic cells or 'blasts' infiltrate the marrow, spleen, lymph nodes, liver and other organs and tissues. The blast cells result from an arrest at a primitive stage in normal cellular differentiation and there is thus a steady accumulation of these long-lived immature cells. Displacement and humoral inhibition of normal marrow cellular elements results in anaemia, neutropenia and thrombocytopenia. Lymphadenopathy is much more a feature of ALL than AML; CNS and testicular involvement are particularly features of ALL.

The history at presentation is usually short and these are nearly always aggressive neoplasms which, untreated, will rapidly result in death. However, in specialist centres approximately 60 per cent of children and 25 per cent of young adults are probably now cured, but the prognosis for older adults is extremely poor.

## Risk factors

Ionising radiation: immunosuppressants and cytotoxic chemotherapy; virus (T cell leukaemia); benzene and toluene; family history; smoking; Down's syndrome; other congenital disorders involving chromosomal fragility or instability, e.g. Klinefelter's syndrome, ataxia telangiectasia, Wiskott-Aldrich syndrome.

## Symptoms and signs

Anaemia
Malaise
Fever
Bone pains
Arthralgia
Hepatosplenomegaly
Lymphadenopathy
Haemorrhage
Stomatitis
Gum infiltration
Peri-anal abscess

# Treatment

### Cytotoxic chemotherapy

For almost all patients initial treatment is now given with curative intent. In the short term this can be considered successful only if remission is obtained, i.e. the absence of all clinical evidence of disease and of detectable leukaemic cells in the peripheral blood and marrow biopsy. The induction of remission involves at least a 2 log (99 per cent) reduction in the total number of leukaemic cells, but at presentation there is usually a total body burden of about $10^{13}$ malignant cells, and therefore further treatment ('consolidation' and, for ALL patients, 'maintenance' treatment for 18 months or more) is necessary.

Combinations of drugs are essential. The drugs used vary according to the type of leukaemia. Rather more aggressive treatment is required for AML. There is considerable variation in the regimens used and most patients are entered into clinical research protocols. The duration of remission induction treatment extends from approximately one week for patients with AML to approximately four weeks for those with ALL. Consolidation and maintenance treatment may last from several months up to 2–3 years. Approximately 10–15 per cent of AML patients will require a second course to secure remission, and 5 per cent remain refractory.

Intravenous chemotherapy does not normally result in drugs crossing the blood-brain barrier in effective concentrations, except for cytosine arabinoside or methotrexate given in high dosage. For patients with ALL, CNS prophylaxis is required because of the high incidence of microscopic CNS involvement. This may be given with either the intrathecal administration of methotrexate plus cranial irradiation, or intrathecal methotrexate plus high dose systemic methotrexate.

Treatment is intensive and complications can be rapidly fatal; supportive care of high standard is therefore essential for success. This includes red cell and platelet transfusions, the prevention and extremely prompt and intensive treatment of bacterial, herpetic and fungal (including pneumocystis) infections, the prevention of uric acid nephropathy with allopurinol and hydration, and the treatment of disseminated intravascular coagulation. Urate nephropathy is a cause of acute renal failure and arises from rapid lysis of large amounts of malignant tissue (tumour lysis syndrome).

Eventual relapse after apparently successful initial treatment is very common. Approximately 30 per cent will already have relapsed at one year, and 40–50 at two years. Further chemotherapy, with the same or different drugs, can induce second remissions but prolonged survival is unusual. Treatment for late relapse is more successful for patients with ALL than AML. Bone marrow transplantation should be considered for relapse in younger patients (see below).

## Radiotherapy

Low-dose whole brain radiation may be given as part of CNS prophylaxis. Treatment is usually completed in two weeks and is very well tolerated in the short term. However, slight long-term intellectual impairment is a risk of CNS prophylaxis in children.

Low dose radiotherapy is occasionally of value in ablating masses of soft tissue disease, e.g. testicular deposits of ALL.

## Leucapheresis

A rapid reduction in the number of circulating leukaemic cells can be achieved by passing the patient's blood through a continuous-flow cell separator. This is very occasionally performed for patients with AML when extremely high cell counts cause an increase in blood viscosity to an extent which interferes with CNS or cardiopulmonary function. However, the viscosity can often be satisfactorily reduced merely by adequate rehydration.

## Marrow transplantation (BMT)

(See separate section in Chapter 7 in Part I.) Where it is feasible, marrow ablative treatment with intensive chemotherapy and whole body irradiation followed by BMT is usually considered the treatment of choice for younger patients with AML in first remission, and for patients with ALL in whom a second remission has been obtained.

Marrow transplantation from an HLA-identical donor appears to be capable of preventing recurrence in about 75 per cent of AML patients when given as consolidation following first remission. The relapse rate is slightly higher for ALL than AML and it increases to approximately 50 per cent for patients transplanted in second remission. However the relapse rate gives no guide to survival because BMT carries a substantial mortality, particularly in centres performing relatively few transplants.

Despite its success in diminishing the likelihood of leukaemic relapse, patients transplanted in first remission continue to experience an approximately 30 per cent likelihood of mortality (rising to approximately 50 per cent for those transplanted in second remission) within 12 months after grafting. This is predominantly due to relapse, but also to complications including pneumonitis, graft versus host disease (GVHD) and CMV infection. Thus BMT in first remission does not yet appear to confer a substantial increase in the chance of long-term survival compared with intensive consolidation chemotherapy, but it does represent the only real chance of cure for adults in second remission. There is evidence to suggest that mild chronic GVHD may be beneficial by exerting an anti-leukaemia effect mediated by allo-T-lymphocytes and, unfortunately, better control of GVHD seems to result in an increased rate of leukaemic relapse. Overall there has been no significant further improvement in survival following BMT for leukaemia during the past decade.

Allogeneic transplantation for AML in first remission is followed by an approximately 50 per cent chance of five-year disease-free survival but this decreases significantly in those over 40 years of age, in whom most complications are more common; BMT is rarely offered to patients over 45 years of age. The median age of patients with AML is over 60 years and less than 20 per cent of patients are younger than 40 years.

Re-infusion of the patient's own bone marrow (autologous as opposed to allogeneic grafting) has been performed for patients with leukaemia in remission as well as for other tumours and there have recently been some encouraging results, despite the very high likelihood that some leukaemic cells are being re-infused into the patient. The number of leukaemic cells re-infused may be insufficient to result in persistent viability of the malignant clone and subsequent clinical relapse. Nevertheless, there are currently under evaluation monoclonal antibody and other techniques designed to purge autologous marrow of leukaemic cells *in vitro*.

## Follow-up

Very close follow-up is usually practised after initial treatment, with frequent peripheral full blood counts to detect early relapse. This is justified because treatment for relapse (particularly first relapse) can be curative and it is reasonable to suppose that the chance of success will be greater if the malignant cell burden is relatively low.

## Practice points

1 The standard of supportive care is crucial to the chance of success. (See Chapters 11 and 12 in Part I.)

2 Adequate hydration and allopurinol should be routine with induction treatment.

3 Septicaemia should be suspected in any unexplained decline in general condition in a neutropenic patient. Hypotension may be present and there may be no fever in patients receiving steroids or in the elderly. A very thorough examination for any source of infection should include the skin (especially injection/catheter sites), oropharynx, mouth and gums, sinuses and peri-anal region. Rectal examination should not be performed as this may cause bacteraemia. Local pain, swelling and inflammation at the site of local infection may be minimal in immunocompromised patients.

4 Immediate treatment of suspected infection with broad-spectrum antibiotics is essential in neutropenic patients, following the taking of blood for culture (aerobic, anaerobic and fungal), swabs of throat and any areas suspicious of infection, an MSU and a chest X-ray.

5 Herpes simplex infection should be suspected in any sore mouth in immunosuppressed patients; classical vesicles are often not seen. Meticulous attention to oral hygiene is important in the prophylaxis of infection. Short-term anti-herpetic prophylaxis with intravenous or oral acyclovir is indicated during leucopenia in herpes simplex seropositive patients (titre >1:10).

6 Infection with *Pneumocystis carinii* should be suspected in breathless patients with pulmonary infiltration who have ALL. It is hardly ever seen in patients with AML. Other fungal infections should also be suspected in febrile patients not rapidly responding to antibiotics and herpetic encephalitis in patients with evidence of intracranial pathology. The empirical administration of amphotericin B is indicated in neutropenic patients with evidence of infection not responding to antibiotics and in whom no causative organism has been discovered.

7 Blood transfusion should be given with platelet cover if the platelet count is below $20 \times 10^9$/litre, otherwise there will be a further decline in the platelet count and a serious risk of haemorrhage. Blood transfusion can increase an already high whole blood viscosity and carry a risk of stroke, particularly in AML patients with very high cell counts.

8 Live vaccines must be avoided both during treatment and subsequently.

9 Long-term survival can occur following admission to an intensive care unit for complications of treatment, frequently involving artificial ventilation for respiratory failure. However, in the presence of dysfunction of an increasing number of organs, failure to recover any marrow function or unresponsive neoplasia the prognosis is extremely poor and further intensive supportive treatment may be inappropriate.

## NOTES

# NOTES

# CHAPTER 26

# Chronic Leukaemias

The annual incidence is about four new cases per 100,000 population. The male/female ratio is 2:1 for chronic lymphocytic leukaemia (CLL) and 1.5:1 for chronic granulocytic leukaemia (CGL), which are the most common types. Approximately 90 per cent of patients with CGL have the Philadelphia chromosomal abnormality within the malignant cells and also in red cell and platelet precursors and some lymphocytes in the marrow. This involves a shortening of the long arm of chromosome number 22, as a result of translocation of genetic material to chromosome number 9. Almost all chronic lymphocytic leukaemias are of B-cell origin.

Very high white cell counts are found in the peripheral blood. There is extensive marrow infiltration but much less interference with normal haemopoiesis than in the acute leukaemias. Lymphadenopathy is extremely common in CLL though rare in CGL; hepatosplenomegaly occurs in both.

The chronic leukaemias can sometimes be extremely indolent, and may be discovered incidentally in asymptomatic patients, particularly CLL. CGL usually runs a biphasic course; the initial relatively indolent chronic phase is followed by a more acute 'accelerated' phase, and entry into acute leukaemia. Most patients will transform within five years of diagnosis. Interestingly, in about 25 per cent of cases these blast cells are apparently of lymphoid origin, indicative of the extent of ancestral marrow cell involvement by the chromosomal abnormality.

Hairy cell leukaemia is an uncommon chronic leukaemia, also of B-lymphocytic origin, which predominantly affects middle-aged men. The leukaemic cells have prominent cytoplasmic projections – 'villi' or 'hairs'. There is marked splenomegaly, and progressive marrow replacement and myelofibrosis lead to pancytopenia.

The majority of non-Hodgkin's lymphomas are also B-lymphoid cell neoplasms. Malignant cells can often be identified in the peripheral blood of these patients and there is thus no fundamental division between CLL and those non-Hodgkin's lymphomas which consist of similar or identical-looking small lymphocytes. The term 'leukaemia' tends to be used when the peripheral blood lymphocyte count exceeds $15 \times 10^9$/litre.

Until relatively recently all chronic leukaemias were considered incurable. Although a small percentage of younger patients (< 50 years) with CGL may now be curable by allogeneic bone marrow transplantation, the median survival overall is 3–4 years. CLL remains incurable but it is a more indolent disease: for those with less bulky and less aggressive disease, survival is comparable with that of the age and sex matched normal population. However, for those presenting with low haemoglobin and platelet counts, the prognosis is worse with a median survival of about only 18 months. For CLL patients overall the median survival is about six years.

Risk factors

Ionising radiation; smoking; family history; possibly welding.

## Symptoms and signs

Malaise
Anaemia
Hepatosplenomegaly
Lymphadenopathy
Abdominal distension
'Dragging' discomfort or pain in left hypochondrium
Fever
Haemorrhage
Bone pain

# Treatment

## Cytotoxic chemotherapy

This is almost always appropriate for patients with CGL as it is relatively non-toxic, often relieves symptoms and probably prolongs median survival by about one year. For patients with CLL there is no firm evidence that treatment prolongs survival. It is usually considered that chemotherapy should be given only for the relief of symptoms or to improve marrow infiltration.

There is no evidence that combinations are better than single agents, except for patients with CGL in accelerated phase or blast crisis. Hydroxyurea is now the drug of choice for chronic phase CGL. It is given orally, either daily or intermittently in a higher dosage every third day. Busulphan was extensively used for CGL but it has been found to compromise the chance of successful bone marrow transplantation.

For CLL oral chlorambucil is the drug most commonly prescribed but other alkylating agents are also effective. It is very well tolerated and is usually given in a low daily dosage, but sometimes intermittently, especially when marrow suppression is a problem.

## Bone marrow transplantation

This should be considered for younger patients with CGL who have an HLA-compatible sibling. There is an approximately 40 per cent chance of five years leukaemia-free survival following BMT in first chronic phase and 25 per cent in accelerated phase. Graft T-cell depletion should not be used as this increases the chance of relapse.

## Corticosteroids

These cause diminution in both neoplastic and normal lymphoid tissue, but otherwise do not cause marrow suppression. This lymphocytolytic effect can be very useful in the management of patients with CLL, especially when there is already marrow suppression. Reduction in tumour bulk can be rapid and steroids are also useful for those patients who develop an auto-immune thrombocytopenia or haemolytic anaemia. However, they should not usually be used continuously because of their long-term side effects, which include a further increase in the risk of infection.

## Radiotherapy

Low dose splenic radiotherapy can be very helpful for some patients with both CGL and CLL. It can achieve a reduction in uncomfortable or painful enlargement, in splenic sequestration of normal blood cells, and also an improvement in the peripheral blood leukaemic cell count as these very radiosensitive cells are irradiated as they pass through the spleen. This systemic benefit may also be seen in the bone marrow and lymph glands.

Low dose local radiotherapy is highly effective in shrinking troublesome CLL lymphadenopathy and in treating other troublesome tissue deposits in patients with both CGL and CLL. Very low dose total body irradiation, usually given over 2–3 weeks, is effective for some patients with chemorefractory CLL.

## Interferon

Alpha interferon gives an 85 per cent response rate in patients with hairy cell leukaemia. No other malignancy is more responsive to interferon, however, the adenosine deaminase inhibitor deoxycoformycin is probably even more effective for these patients.

## Splenectomy

This is the initial treatment of choice for hairy cell leukaemia. It is also occasionally indicated where there is persistent excessive splenic sequestration of normal blood cells (hypersplenism), auto-immune anaemia orthrombocytopenia, or massive unresponsive splenomegaly causing severe symptoms. Patients should receive pneumococcal vaccine at least two weeks before surgery and long-term penicillin prophylaxis afterwards, if tolerated.

## Leucapheresis

This is occasionally indicated for patients with blood hyperviscosity due to both CGL and CLL. Hyperviscosity is more common in CGL as myeloid cells are larger and more rigid than lymphoid cells.

## Follow-up

Prolonged specialist supervision is appropriate for these patients, involving regular assessments of response and full blood count monitoring. The value of out-patient attendance may be debatable when the disease enters a terminal phase. Although repeated blood transfusions can improve symptoms markedly in the short term it is a matter of judgement how long such support should continue. Once started it is often difficult to discontinue.

## Practice points

1 Supportive care includes the prompt treatment of infections since patients with CLL, like those with acute leukaemia (but to a lesser extent), are immunosuppressed both by their disease and its treatment. Immunosuppression is not usually a problem in patients with CGL.
2 Prophylactic allopurinol should be given to prevent urate nephropathy.
3 Live vaccines must be avoided.
4 Significant whole blood hyperviscosity can occur in patients with CGL and very high cell counts. It may cause bleeding, retinopathy, brain dysfunction, cardiac failure and priapism. Blood transfusion can produce a dangerous further increase.

# NOTES

# CHAPTER 27

# Myeloma

The annual incidence is approximately four per 100,000 population. The male/female ratio is 1:1. Myeloma is a malignant monoclonal accumulation of plasma cells, which are the fully differentiated antibody-producing 'end-cells' of the B-lymphocyte lineage. However, the neoplastic proliferation also involves precursor cells at an earlier stage in the lineage: myeloma should not be considered purely as a malignancy of plasma cells.

Myeloma is almost always a systemic disease, hence the term *multiple myeloma*. It almost always involves marrow and surrounding bone. Very occasionally bone deposits do appear to be truly solitary, and the very rare 'extramedullary plasmacytomas' which usually arise within lymphatic tissue in the pharynx or paranasal sinuses are usually solitary. In multiple myeloma the presence of multiple osteolytic lesions is typical. Osteoclasts are activated and osteoblasts are inhibited by the malignant cells, and usually there is very little attempt to repair the damage. Isotope bone scans and serum alkaline phosphatase concentrations are thus quite often normal.

Multiple myeloma almost invariably produces monoclonal immunoglobulins (paraproteins), which are detectable in the serum. Usually whole immunoglobulin molecules are produced and about 50 per cent of patients produce IgG and 25 per cent IgA. In about 70 per cent of cases light chain moieties (Bence-Jones protein) are produced, usually in addition to whole immunoglobulin molecules, but in approximately 20 per cent of patients only light chains are produced. Because of the smaller size of the light chain molecules Bence-Jones protein is detectable in the urine, although it may sometimes be difficult to detect unless the urine is concentrated. The malignant plasma cell proliferation results in a suppression both of normal antibody production and of normal marrow function. Deposition of light chains in soft tissues (amyloidosis) occurs in about 10 per cent of patients, affecting principally the kidneys, tongue, gastro-intestinal tract, nervous system and heart.

The presence of a serum paraprotein is not sufficient by itself to diagnose multiple myeloma. Monoclonal paraproteins can also be detected in other conditions, notably non-Hodgkin's lymphoma. About 20 per cent of people with serum paraproteins have a 'benign monoclonal gammopathy', where there is no increase over a five-year period, no evidence of abnormal plasma cells in the marrow, and no evidence of osteolysis. Two of these three criteria are necessary for the diagnosis of multiple myeloma. However, some patients with supposed benign monoclonal gammopathy do subsequently develop frank multiple myeloma, suggesting a continuous spectrum.

The majority of patients with a supposedly solitary bone plasmacytoma ultimately develop widespread disease but a minority are cured, and substantially more than 50 per cent of those with solitary extra-osseous plasmacytoma. For the much greater number of patients with multiple myeloma there is no prospect of cure. With treatment the median survival for those with multiple myeloma is 2–3 years: only about 20 per cent of patients are alive at five years. The outlook is worse for patients with more extensive disease (who usually have higher serum paraprotein concentrations and anaemia), those producing IgA paraprotein (as opposed to IgG) and Bence-Jones protein only, and for those with renal impairment. The prognosis is also poor for patients with high serum $\beta$-2 microglobulin concentrations, but levels $<5$ µg/ml are usually associated with long survival. Elevation of these levels can, however, occur as a result of renal impairment and formulae are available for the prognostic interpretation of raised levels when this is present.

Risk factors

Ionising radiation; family history.

## Symptoms and signs

Bone pain
Pathological fracture
Anaemia
Symptoms of hypercalcaemia and renal failure
Fever due to infection
Bleeding
Hyperviscosity syndrome (confusion, lethargy, visual disturbance, bleeding tendency)

# Treatment

### Cytotoxic chemotherapy

Treatment of multiple myeloma is usually given with the intent of prolonging life and relieving symptoms. Cure has not hitherto been considered a possibility, but it now appears that allo-bone marrow transplantation after disease stabilisation can result in long-term survival for some patients.

Cytotoxic chemotherapy is usually the mainstay of treatment and the serial estimation of serum paraprotein concentrations allows sensitive monitoring of progress. Most commonly a single oral alkylating agent, melphalan or cyclophosphamide, is prescribed continuously, or intermittently at higher dosage. The response rate may be increased by the addition of prednisolone, although the evidence is conflicting, but it does not seem to have much impact on survival. Approximately 35 per cent of patients respond to melphalan alone, and 50 per cent with the addition of prednisolone. A fall in the paraprotein concentration to <10 per cent of the starting value characterises a favourable prognostic group in whom median survival may be further prolonged by about a year.

Although maintenance treatment with melphalan and prednisolone after disease stabilisation for four months delays relapse, there is no evidence that it improves survival. About 50 per cent of patients not given maintenance treatment will respond to the same treatment again on relapse. More intensive and toxic regimens using high dose melphalan or drug combinations may slightly improve survival and may be considered justifiable for younger patients (< 65 years), but there is as yet no clear evidence of significant advantage over conventional treatment with melphalan and prednisolone.

## Radiotherapy

Myeloma is very radiosensitive and palliative low dose radiotherapy is highly successful for localised bone pain. Intermediate dose radiotherapy, given with curative intent, is the treatment of choice for solitary plasmacytoma. Very low dose whole body irradiation given over about three weeks as a systemic treatment for multiple myeloma has comparable efficacy to chemotherapy, but marrow suppression is more profound.

## Interferon

Alpha interferon has some anti-myeloma activity but is usually less effective and more toxic than standard chemotherapy. It may possibly have a rôle when given as maintenance after disease stabilisation.

## Diphosphonates

These may be useful in inhibiting osteoclastic activity in patients with or without hypercalcaemia. (See section on hypercalcaemia in Chapter 13 in Part I.)

## **Follow-up**

Chemotherapy should be monitored closely for response and toxicity. It should be continued until the maximum effect is achieved and a plateau is reached for three to four months in the paraprotein concentration. There is no survival advantage in continuing treatment further but continued follow-up is usually justified since a substantial minority will respond on relapse to the same or alternative chemotherapy.

## Practice points

1 The prompt and successful treatment of serious complications is particularly important at presentation since this may permit benefit from cytotoxic treatment directed against the malignancy itself. Such complications include pain, infection, hypercalcaemia, renal failure and hyperviscosity.

2 Prophylactic allopurinol should be given during the first couple of months of treatment to prevent urate nephropathy.

3 High fluid intake ($\geqslant$ 3 litres per day) is important to reduce the risk of renal failure and hypercalcaemia, particularly those with detectable urinary light chains.

4 Maintenance of mobility is important in the prophylaxis of bone demineralisation and hypercalcaemia, and is often made easier by achieving satisfactory relief of pain. However, patients should be warned about their brittle bones and the hazards of falling.

5 In about one per cent of patients no paraprotein can be detected due to the undifferentiated nature of the plasma cells.

**NOTES**

# NOTES

# CHAPTER 28

# Non-Hodgkin's Lymphoma

The annual incidence is approximately eight per 100,000 population. In almost all cases the cell of origin is a lymphocyte, and the neoplastic change is usually in the B-lymphocyte lineage although some lymphomas arise from T-lymphocytes and histiocytes. The malignant lymphocytes correspond to varying stages in normal lymphocyte differentiation and maturation. At one end of the spectrum the neoplastic accumulation is of small lymphocytes which normally exhibit very little mitotic activity. At the other there is an accumulation of much larger lymphocytes which have the ability to produce (but not necessarily secrete) immunoglobulins and which frequently undergo mitosis. These are respectively examples of 'low-grade' and 'high-grade' lymphomas, the latter being far more aggressive. In between are lymphomas classified as being of 'intermediate grade'.

The cells of some low and intermediate grade lymphomas retain the ability of some normal lymphocytes to form follicles (follicular lymphomas) whilst in others the lymphocytes have lost this ability (diffuse lymphomas). Most diffuse lymphomas (but not those composed of small lymphocytes) are more aggressive than follicular lymphomas. In general the larger the neoplastic lymphocytes the more aggressive (the higher grade) the lymphoma. There is a continuous spectrum and many lymphomas contain mixtures of neoplastic cells corresponding to different stages of normal differentiation.

In contrast to Hodgkin's disease there is overall a substantially greater tendency for simultaneous widespread involvement, rather than for contiguous lymph node spread. Paradoxically, low-grade lymphomas have an even greater tendency to be generalised than high-grade tumours. However, some low-grade lymphomas are extremely indolent and may even undergo spontaneous partial regression from time to time. High-grade lymphomas, being composed of cells with considerable mitotic activity, tend to increase in size rapidly. After a period of many months or some years low-grade lymphomas may sometimes transform to a higher grade.

The most common manifestation is lymphadenopathy, localised or generalised. Involvement of the bone marrow and spleen is very common, particularly in low-grade lymphomas (approximately 95 per cent) and there can also be involvement of liver, skin, mucosa, gut, bone, thyroid, testes and CNS. With low-grade lymphomas there is sometimes an overt neoplastic lymphocytosis in the peripheral blood and thus no real distinction from chronic lymphatic leukaemia. Mycosis fungoides is a T-lymphocyte lymphoma which primarily involves skin, usually diffusely. At a later stage lymph node and visceral involvement can occur.

Although the majority of patients respond to treatment even 'complete' responses are often followed by relapse. Another paradox is that 'cure' of low-grade lymphomas is extremely rare: although they are often compatible with several years of good-quality life the disease nearly always re-asserts itself at some stage if the patient lives long enough. The usual survival for patients with low-grade lymphomas is 5–10 years. In contrast, about 25 per cent of those with intermediate and high-grade lymphomas are cured and the chance of cure rises considerably above 50 per cent where the disease appears to be truly localised; for patients with high-grade lymphomas who are not cured prolonged survival is unusual. Overall, non-Hodgkin's lymphoma carries a substantially worse prognosis than Hodgkin's disease and it is particularly poor for those with substantial tumour bulk.

## Risk factors

Immunosuppression (including immune deficiency syndromes, organ transplantation, auto-immune diseases and AIDS); coeliac disease; viral infection (T-cell lymphoma [HTLV I] and Burkitt's lymphoma [EBV]); phenytoin; ionising radiation; cytotoxic chemotherapy; possibly phenoxyherbicides.

**Symptoms and signs**

Painless rubbery lymphadenopathy
Hepatosplenomegaly
Waldeyer's ring involvement (tonsils and nasopharynx)
Skin plaques
Extranodal masses at other sites (e.g. orbit)
Fever
Night sweats
Weight loss
Pruritus
Anaemia
Superior vena caval obstruction

# Treatment

### Radical

Surgery

The role of surgery is usually limited to establishing the diagnosis. Excision of masses of gastrointestinal lymphoma is advisable, however, as treatment with chemotherapy or radiotherapy may be followed by perforation.

Radiotherapy

These are very radiosensitive neoplasms although high-grade lymphomas sometimes require quite high doses. Radiotherapy is frequently curative for the relatively uncommon patients with apparently localised tumours. Most of these have intermediate or high-grade lymphomas, frequently involving the head and neck.

Cytotoxic chemotherapy

Treatment with curative intent is appropriate only for those with intermediate or high-trade lymphomas and the very small number of those with low-grade lymphomas that still appear localised after intensive staging investigations. Combinations of drugs are essential for cure and if an early complete clinical remission is not obtained success is unlikely. Some types of lymphoma carry a higher risk of CNS involvement, and CNS prophylaxis with intrathecal chemotherapy with or without cranial irradiation may be indicated.

## Marrow transplantation

Marrow ablative treatment followed by allografting or autografting is an experimental approach for younger patients with intermediate or high-grade lymphomas. It may be considered for those who are in second remission or relapse after initially successful treatment, and even for those with very poor prognostic features who have just presented; the chance of long-term survival, however, appears to be very low.

## Palliative

### Radiotherapy

Low dose irradiation is very useful for troublesome masses of low-grade lymphomas even though the disease is generalised. Low-dose whole body irradiation over two to three weeks is often effective for disseminated low-grade lymphomas, but is usually more marrow suppressive than chemotherapy. Skin plaques of mycosis fungoides respond very well to superficial low dose irradiation. When this disease is widespread but still very superficial a specialised technique of total skin irradiation using low energy electrons can achieve excellent results. PUVA has also been used successfully for this condition.

### Cytotoxic chemotherapy

Relatively gentle chemotherapy with single agents, e.g. oral chlorambucil, or non-aggressive combinations plus or minus prednisolone are often very effective for low-grade lymphoma but the full effect of treatment may not be seen for several months. Treatment for most patients with low-grade lymphomas may be approached in the same way as for B-cell chronic lymphocytic leukaemia and it is reasonable to withhold treatment when the disease is indolent, not threatening any vital structure and causing no troublesome symptoms.

## Interferon

This has shown useful activity against low-grade lymphomas but is more toxic than single agent chemotherapy.

## Follow-up

Long-term out-patient follow-up is probably justified for the majority of patients after apparently successful initial treatment since relapse is common but can quite often be effectively treated: cure following relapse is very unusual but useful palliation or a further remission can be achieved with further chemotherapy or radiotherapy.

## Practice points

1 Patients considered potentially suitable for radical treatment should be thoroughly staged whenever time allows. Staging investigations will include liver function tests, serum immunoglobulins, marrow aspirate and trephine, examination of oro- and naso-pharynx and CT scans of chest and abdomen. Staging laparotomy is no longer performed in the UK but remains common in the USA.

2 CSF examination for protein concentration and post-centrifugation immuno-cytology should be considered in patients with high-grade lymphoma involving marrow or bone and it should be performed whenever there is any clinical feature suggestive of CNS involvement.

3 Patients with bulky disease should be well hydrated (3 litres/m$^2$/day) and receive prophylactic allopurinol prior to and during initial treatment.

4 Increasingly aggressive chemotherapeutic regimens are being used in radical treatment and as with acute leukaemia the standard of supportive care is crucial to the avoidance of treatment-related death.

5 Impaired immunity is extremely common in these

patients. The approach to the prophylaxis and treatment of infections adopted in the management of acute leukaemia is appropriate for patients receiving aggressive cytotoxic chemotherapy. Live vaccines are contra-indicated in all patients.

6  Deep vein thrombosis and pulmonary embolism is a potential complication of cytotoxic chemotherapy for non-Hodgkin's lymphoma, probably at least partly due to the combination of pelvic disease with dehydration.

7  A stable residual mass after cytotoxic chemotherapy judged to have been otherwise successful does not necessarily contain any residual malignant cells. In the abdomen fine needle aspiration should be considered, but it is usually reasonable to follow closely such masses clinically and radiologically without surgical exploration.

**NOTES**

# NOTES

# CHAPTER 29

# Oesophageal Carcinoma

The incidence is approximately eight per 100,000 population annually and the male/female ratio 3:2. Squamous carcinomas constitute 90 per cent of the total: most of the remainder are adenocarcinomas and arise at the lower end. Most tumours present at an advanced stage and there is a high incidence of both local and metastatic spread. If the tumour length is >5 cm there is only a 10 per cent chance that the disease is confined to the oesophagus. Potentially curative treatment with either radiotherapy or surgery should be considered for patients in good general health who have relatively small tumours with no evidence of spread outside the oesophagus. Overall only about 20 per cent of patients survive one year and only about 5 per cent are cured, but the outlook is slightly better for selected patients with small tumours treated radically.

### Risk factors

Smoking and alcohol, particularly the combination; Plummer Vinson syndrome; familial tylosis; possibly achalasia, tannin, and hot drinks.

### Spread

Submucosally up and down via lymphatics; mediastinal, supraclavicular and diaphragmatic nodes; lungs and liver. The lack of an oesophageal serosal covering probably facilitates early invasion of adjacent mediastinal structures.

## Symptoms and signs

Dysphagia, initially worse for solids than liquids
Weight loss
Pain on swallowing, sometimes radiating to back
Cough on swallowing (tracheo-oesophageal fistula)
Supraclavicular lymphadenopathy

# Treatment

### Radical

### Surgery

This is preferred for apparently localised tumours of the lower oesophagus. For carcinomas of the middle third there seems to be little to choose between surgery or radiotherapy. A wide resection margin is important, ideally 12 cm from macroscopically detectable growth. Several procedures are practised, using various combinations of cervical, thoracic and abdominal approaches. The oesophagus can be removed via cervical and abdominal incisions; a thoracotomy is not necessarily essential. Laparotomy not only enables mobilisation of the stomach, but allows assessment of the extent of lymph node involvement. If there is obvious involvement of the upper abdominal nodes it is highly debatable whether radical surgery should be proceeded with. Continuity may be re-established by bringing the stomach up to the proximal resection margin, or by using a segment of bowel.

Radical surgery is a very major procedure. Recovery may often be prolonged and the hospital mortality varies from five to 30 per cent indicating the necessity for careful patient selection.

### Radiotherapy

This is preferred for carcinomas of the upper third of the oesophagus, and often offered for middle third lesions; it will usually last from 4-6 weeks. Radiation oesophagitis is inevitable and it is very important to maintain adequate nutrition and hydration. It is otherwise usually fairly well tolerated although side-effects include stricture, radiation pneumonitis and very rarely spinal cord damage.

## Combined modality

Many combinations of surgery, pre- or post-operative radiotherapy, and cytotoxic chemotherapy have been tried, but none has been proven to improve the chance of cure over surgery or radiotherapy alone.

## Palliative

### Surgery

Intubation to relieve dysphagia is the generally preferred palliative procedure. It can also be useful for patients with oesophago-respiratory fistula. It is most easily performed endoscopically although some tubes require pulling down via a gastrostomy. Relief of symptoms is immediate and patients can usually leave hospital relatively quickly. However there is a risk of perforation and high mortality rates have been reported from some hospitals. Bougienage can be dangerous and is rarely employed. By-pass procedures using stomach or bowel are occasionally used but for most patients this is over-vigorous. There is now considerable enthusiasm for palliating dysphagia by laser destruction of the endophytic tumour. However, significant complicaitons occur in about 25 per cent of patients, especially when repeated courses are given. These can be severe and fatal, e.g. perforation and aorto-oesophageal fistula. Another recently described technique is the induction of tumour necrosis by the direct injection of 10–15 ml of dehydrated ethanol.

### Radiotherapy

Palliative external radiotherapy, commonly given over a couple of weeks, is generally well tolerated but not as effective in relieving dysphagia as intubation. Using a remote afterloading machine intracavitary radiotherapy with a tube containing radioactive caesium is now possible without incurring a radiation hazard to staff; this has been reported to be quick, effective and well tolerated.

## Cytotoxic chemotherapy

Response rates are very low and this has no place in routine management.

## Follow-up

Failure after radical treatment with either radiotherapy or surgery cannot be salvaged. There is thus no justification for close follow-up, and any further treatment should await the onset of symptoms.

## Practice points

1 Overt metastatic disease must be excluded prior to radical treatment. Supraclavicular fossae examination, chest radiography and liver function tests are essential, and a CT scan of the chest will often give further useful information.
2 Recurrence of dysphagia can be due to benign post-surgical or post-radiation stricture.

## NOTES

# NOTES

# CHAPTER 30

# Ovarian Carcinoma

The incidence is approximately 16 per 100,000 women annually and is thus comparable with cervical carcinoma. Ovarian carcinomas very often grow to a considerable size before causing symptoms, however, and only 10 per cent of patients present with tumour confined to one ovary. They are often bilateral, break through the ovarian capsule and spread into the peritoneal cavity at an early stage. About one-third of patients with disease macroscopically confined to the pelvis have unrecognised disease spread. Approximately two-thirds of patients present with overt peritoneal metastases and this tumour is responsible for substantially the greatest number of deaths from gynaecological malignancy.

All tumours of the germinal epithelium have a tendency to cyst formation, although increasing malignancy results in an increasingly solid component. They are classified as mucinous, serous or endometrioid according to the contents of the cysts and the histological appearance of the cells lining them. Mucinous carcinomas tend to be better differentiated and carry a better prognosis. In about 15 per cent of tumours differentiation between classification as benign or malignant is very difficult: the epithelial cells may look malignant but there may be no evidence of invasion of the underlying stroma. Such tumours are classified as being of borderline malignancy and carry a good prognosis.

The overall cure rate for ovarian carcinoma is about 25 per cent. For Stage I disease (macroscopically confined to one or both ovaries) the five-year survival is approximately 65 per cent; for Stage II disease (confined to pelvis) approximately 40 per cent; for Stage III (intraperitoneal dissemination) and Stage IV disease (liver or extra-abdominal involvement) approximately 5 per cent. For those with advanced disease capable of receiving optimal surgery and chemotherapy the five-year survival rate can rise to as much as 15–20 per cent, but almost all will eventually relapse.

## Risk factors

Nulliparity; no history of oral contraception; infertility; previous breast carcinoma; gonadal dysgenesis; Peutz Jegher's syndrome; ionising radiation; possibly asbestos and high lactose (yogurt and cottage cheese) consumption.

## Spread

Direct spread occurs to other pelvic viscera but this tumour has a marked tendency to spread extensively trans-coelomically. Diffuse peritoneal and omental deposits are common and these are quite frequently found on the undersurface of the diaphragm. Lymphatic spread occurs to para-aortic, pelvic, mediastinal and supraclavicular nodes. Blockage of mediastinal lymphatics by tumour is an important contributory factor to the frequent development of ascites. Pleural involvement is also common and blood-borne spread is principally to the lungs and liver.

## Symptoms and signs

Vague non-specific abdominal symptoms
Upper and lower abdominal/pelvic pain
Abdominal distension
Post menopausal bleeding
Urinary frequency
Constipation
Ascites
Pelvic mass
Pleural effusion
Hepatomegaly
Supraclavicular lymphadenopathy

# Treatment

## Radical

### Surgery

For ovarian carcinoma total abdominal hysterectomy and bilateral salpingo-oophorectomy is the minimum initial treatment of choice for patients other than those with very extensive disease. A thorough attempt should be made to discover the true extent of the disease within the whole abdominal cavity. Any ascitic fluid should be sent for cytology and if there is no ascites about 300 ml of normal saline should be instilled into the peritoneal cavity and the washings sent for cytology.

When there is extensive disease, ideally as much tumour as possible should be removed, which may involve removal of much of the omentum. Such 'de-bulking' surgery improves the chance of subsequent benefit from cytotoxic chemotherapy. It requires a vertical incision and ideally should be undertaken by a gynaecologist with specialised expertise.

### Radiotherapy

Whole abdominal and pelvic external radiotherapy has been practised as a post-surgical adjuvant treatment for patients with Stage II and unfavourable Stage I tumours. The whole abdominal cavity does not tolerate radiation well and thus such treatment must be given slowly and to only a relatively low dose. It has been claimed to improve survival but the evidence from different studies is conflicting. It is possible that platinum-containing cytotoxic chemotherapy may be equally or more effective although no randomised trial has been reported. The intraperitoneal instillation of radioactive isotopes (colloidal phosphorus or gold) has been advocated as an adjuvant treatment for patients with unfavourable Stage I disease but there has not yet been convincing evidence of benefit.

## Cytotoxic chemotherapy

Ovarian carcinoma is relatively responsive to cytotoxic chemotherapy, response rates being as high as 70 per cent for some combinations. Cytotoxic chemotherapy can undoubtedly prolong survival for some patients and may be capable of contributing to cure for a very small percentage. It should be considered for all patients with residual disease after surgery and for all patients with Stage I or II disease who have not had a bilateral salpingo-oophorectomy.

The results tend to be much better where the diameter of residual tumour deposits after surgery is under 2 cm. Cisplatinum has been the most effective single agent but it is toxic; its analogue, carboplatin, is much better tolerated and may be equally as effective. Response rates are higher with drug combinations than with platinum as a single agent, but they have not been demonstrated to improve survival since toxicity is also higher.

Intraperitoneal chemotherapy is at present under evaluation; it achieves higher drug concentrations in the peritoneal cavity than in the plasma, and offers the prospect of improving the therapeutic ratio, although useful penetration beneath the peritoneal surface is probably limited.

## Palliative

### Surgery

Patients who remain in good general condition but who have re-accumulating ascites may benefit from a LeVeen shunt. This is a relatively quick and simple procedure where a subcutaneously-tunnelled tube joins the peritoneal cavity and superior vena cava; it is sometimes followed by transient fever or mild heart failure.

Pleurodesis may be considered for recurrent pleural effusion.

### Cytotoxic chemotherapy

Response rates of 40–50 per cent are achievable with single alkylating agents (e.g. oral melphalan or chlorambucil and intramuscular thiotepa), and these are usually very well tolerated. Such treatment is often suitable for frail or elderly patients and very occasionally is followed by long-term (more than five years) survival for patients presenting with advanced disease.

## Endocrine therapy

Occasional responses have been reported with progestogens. Although the chance of an objective response is low ($\leq 10$ per cent) progestogens can sometimes improve the patient's general well-being.

## Follow-up

'Second-look' surgery for patients in clinical remission after chemotherapy is sometimes performed with the aim of defining those patients who have no residual macroscopic tumour, and of resecting any persistent tumour in the remainder. A recent randomised trial has, however, failed to show that it confers any survival benefit.

There is no evidence to suggest that cure is possible for patients who do not respond to initial treatment or for those who relapse after it.

## Practice points

1 Laparotomy in patients with ovarian carcinoma should ideally be performed by those experienced in the thorough assessment of disease extent and in the debulking of extensive disease.
2 Since widespread ovarian carcinoma quite often responds well to non-toxic chemotherapy, an ultrasound ovarian scan may be a justifiable investigation in women presenting with metastatic carcinoma from an unknown primary site, particularly those with ascites and/or pleural effusions.

# NOTES

# CHAPTER 31

# Pancreatic Cancer

In the western world the incidence of pancreatic cancer has trebled during the past 30 years and is now approximately 12 per 100,000 population annually, with equal distribution between males and females. About 95 per cent of malignant pancreatic tumours are carcinomas arising from the exocrine parts of the gland. The endocrine islet cells give rise to both benign and malignant tumours; the malignant tumours are usually very well differentiated and unless there are metastases present it can be difficult to distinguish between them.

The majority of carcinomas arise in the head of the pancreas where they can easily cause obstruction of pancreatic and common bile ducts. These are very aggressive tumours and only 10 per cent or less of patients present with disease confined to the pancreas. The median survival is about six months with the survival at one and five years only 10 per cent and 3 per cent respectively. The five-year survival for the small minority who have resectable tumours is only 10–15 per cent.

Islet cell tumours are by contrast usually relatively indolent and carry a much better prognosis. They commonly secrete hormones, including insulin, glucagon, gastrin and vaso-active intestinal polypeptide, depending on the cell of origin. These can give rise to a variety of effects, of which the Zollinger-Ellison syndrome (severe peptic ulceration from excessive gastrin-stimulated hyperacidity) and hypoglycaemia from insulinoma are best known.

Risk factors

Smoking; diabetes.

Spread

For pancreatic carcinomas both local invasion and more distant spread are very common. The former is to the duodenum, stomach, retroperitoneal tissues and coeliac plexus and the latter occurs toloco-regional lymph nodes, liver and peritoneum. Islet cell tumours spread principally to lymph nodes and liver.

## Symptoms and signs

   Upper abdominal pain, often radiating to back and
   occasionally relieved by sitting forward
   Jaundice
   Pruritus
   Weight loss
   Nausea/vomiting
   Hepatomegaly
   Palpable gallbladder
   Abdominal mass
   Supraclavicular lymphadenopathy
   Symptoms of diabetes
   Ascites
   Migratory thrombophlebitis

Endocrine effects from islet cell tumours:

Dizziness, confusion, epilepsy, coma (insulin)
Severe peptic ulceration, haemorrhage, perforation (gastrin)
Watery diarrhoea (vasoactive intestinal polypeptide)
Hyperglycaemia and a migratory necrolytic erythematous rash (glucagon)

# Treatment

## Radical

### Surgery

Excision offers the only chance of cure and should be considered for the small number of patients presenting with localised disease. Only about 15 per cent of those thought to have localised disease pre-operatively are, however, found to have resectable tumours. The standard (Whipple's) operation involves removal of the duodenum, gastric antrum, distal bile duct and gall bladder. The operative mortality rate is 15–20 per cent and the risk of severe complications including fistulae and haemorrhage even higher. More radical procedures have been advocated but are of unproven value.

### Radiotherapy

The upper abdomen does not tolerate radiotherapy well and there is very little place for this treatment modality in routine management. There is some evidence that adjuvant radiotherapy combined with cytotoxic chemotherapy may slightly improve median survival, but at a cost of considerable additional morbidity. In Japan and the USA there is some enthusiasm for intra-operative radiotherapy delivered to the tumour bed at the time of surgical exploration, but the value of this approach has also yet to be established.

## Palliative

### Surgery

Most patients are found to have unresectable disease, but since biliary obstruction is extremely common it is usually considered advisable to perform a biliary by-pass procedure at laparotomy. This may be either a cholecystojejunostomy or a choledochojejunostomy; a gastroenterostomy may be offered to relieve obstruction in the duodenal region. These procedures are usually relatively well tolerated.

Biliary obstruction can usually be relieved by the insertion of a biliary stent endoscopically or percutaneously, the former usually being safer and more successful.

Hepatic artery embolisation can provide very useful palliation of local and endocrine symptoms arising from liver metastases from islet cell tumours.

Gastrectomy has an important place in the management of Zollinger-Ellison syndrome, particularly for those patients not responding to $H_2$-receptor antagonist drugs. The substantial majority of patients with this syndrome have unresectable tumours.

### Radiotherapy

This has a very limited palliative rôle: radiotherapy is poorly tolerated in the upper abdomen.

### Cytotoxic chemotherapy

Response rates are low and this has no place in the routine management of carcinomas.

Streptozotocin is a cytotoxic drug with a special affinity for islet cells. About 50 per cent of patients with insulinomas respond to this drug and about 15 per cent experience very substantial benefit. Nausea, vomiting and renal toxicity are common.

### Other drugs

Somatostatin analogue produces substantial suppression of hormone secretion in about 75 per cent of pancreatic endocrine tumours, often lasting several months and sometimes longer.

Interferon also has some activity against pancreatic endocrine tumours. $H_2$-receptor antagonists are highly effective in the management of Zollinger-Ellison syndrome. Diazoxide suppresses insulin release from islet cells and is useful for patients with inoperable insulinomas.

## Follow-up

There is no chance of curative salvage following failed initial surgery. In the absence of symptoms there is usually no good justification for regular hospital attendance.

## Practice point

Patients with severe upper abdominal pain frequently benefit from a coeliac plexus block.

## NOTES

# CHAPTER 32

# Prostatic Carcinoma

There are about 35 new cases per 100,000 males per annum, almost all being adenocarcinomas which usually arise from peripheral glandular tissue. This tumour has some features in common with breast carcinoma; both are hormonally responsive, both have a high incidence of lymphatic and blood-borne metastases, and both can have a very long natural history. The majority of prostate carcinomas are, however, indolent neoplasms with little capacity for local or distant spread, and therefore go undiagnosed. Microscopic occult carcinomas are found in 15 per cent of middle-aged men at autopsy and in 60 per cent of those in the eighth decade. Many small tumours may have little propensity for further growth and it is difficult to evaluate radical local treatments for them, particularly as those growths which are more aggressive have a high tendency to produce distant metastases. Metastatic spread seems to occur only from tumours greater than about 4 ml in volume, and this size is attained by less than 15 per cent of carcinomas discovered incidentally at autopsy. However, only about 10 per cent of clinically detected carcinomas are localised to the prostate; the great majority have extended outside the capsule at the time of diagnosis and about 30 per cent of these will already have distant metastases evident on a bone scan.

The overall relative five-year survival rate is about 35 per cent. Survival is highest for men in late middle age and falls with advancing age. The prognosis is also significantly worse for the small minority of men diagnosed under the age of 55. However, as with breast carcinoma, five-year survival is far from being equivalent to cure. For patients with tumours apparently localised to the prostate, survival at five years exceeds 75 per cent, but falls to about 50 per cent at ten years and 35 per cent at 15 years.

### Risk factor

Industrial exposure to ionising radiation.

### Spread

Local spread to seminal vesicles is very common and the degree of differentiation is correlated with the propensity to metastasise. About 25 per cent of patients with clinically localised tumours which are well differentiated have pelvic lymph node involvement, compared with over 50 per cent of those which are poorly differentiated. Distant spread to bone is particularly common, principally via Batson's paravertebral venous plexus to the proximal femora, pelvis, vertebrae and ribs. Bone metastases are usually osteosclerotic due to a predominance of osteoblastic over osteolytic activity, and thus the incidence of pathological fracture is relatively low.

### Symptoms and signs

Prostatism
Pain from bone metastases is frequently the first symptom
Many patients are asymptomatic and the diagnosis is suspected at routine rectal examination
Supraclavicular lymphadenopathy

# Treatment

### Radical

#### Surgery

There has been considerable enthusiasm for radical local treatment with surgery or radiotherapy for patients with palpable but small tumours apparently confined within the prostatic capsule, and for radical radiotherapy for slightly more extensive but still apparently localised tumours. However, there remains uncertainty concerning the natural history of the disease, particularly the smaller tumours. There is also a dearth of randomised controlled studies, especially those of sufficient duration, bearing in mind the potentially very long natural history of this tumour. The real value of radical local treatments compared with an expectant approach or hormonal manipulation therefore remains unproven; there is, however, widespread acceptance that, on the evidence that is available, radical treatments may be justifiably offered to some patients.

Some patients have no palpable tumour, but are discovered incidentally to have a prostatic carcinoma as a result of histological examination of curettings from transurethral resection or following a simple prostatectomy performed for supposedly benign hypertrophy: there is widespread acceptance that no further treatment is indicated. There is a less than 10 per cent chance of subsequent evidence of tumour activity, and the mortality from cancer in one large series of such patients was only 2 per cent.

Radical prostatectomy has been particularly popular in the USA and in mainland Europe, but not in the United Kingdom. It is usually offered only to patients with tumours presumed to be confined within the prostatic capsule. The prostate, capsule, seminal vesicles and vas deferens are all removed and virtually all patients are rendered impotent. Other adverse sequelae include incontinence, ureteric damage and recto-vesical fistula.

## Radiotherapy

Most radical radiotherapy has been given with external beams. Patients are often offered radical radiotherapy for tumours that are a little larger than those considered treatable by surgery. For tumours of the same stage the results appear to be comparable with those of surgery. Acute radiation effects on the bladder and rectum are inevitable and 10–20 per cent of patients experience troublesome chronic symptomatology from the late effects on these structures,

including haemorrhage from telangiectatic radiation proctitis; impotence only occurs in about one-third of patients.
Patients should be treated with a full bladder, which helps to
push the small bowel out of the treatment volume.

Interstitial irradiation has been advocated in an attempt to
reduce side effects: radioactive sources such as $^{125}$I seeds or
$^{198}$Au grains may be inserted into the prostate via suprapubic
or perineal approaches. Impotence appears to be less common
than with external irradiation, but long-term efficacy is not
yet established.

## Palliative

### Surgery

Transurethral resection provides rapid relief of obstructive
symptoms although these can also be improved, but more
slowly, by endocrine manipulation.

Bilateral orchidectomy is the yardstick with which other
hormonal manipulations should be compared. It is usually
considered that a subcapsular removal is adequate, and if
necessary this can be done under local anaesthesia. This
operation leaves palpable intrascrotal masses, nevertheless
the main drawback is the psychological impact of castration;
many patients are therefore reluctant to accept it. The reduction in testosterone secretion results in a diminution of libido
and, to a lesser extent, also in potency for some patients.
Another common side effect is hot flushes. Painful gynaecomastia can occur after orchidectomy but this is less common
than with oestrogens. Orchidectomy does not carry the cardiovascular hazards of oestrogen therapy, and there is no
problem with drug compliance. As with other hormonal manoeuvres about 75 per cent of patients experience symptomatic
improvement. Half of these will relapse within two years and
less than 10 per cent survive ten years. Only about 5 per cent
of patients benefit from orchidectomy following stilboestrol
failure.

Some pain relief is seen in about two-thirds of patients with
relapsing advanced bone disease following hypophysectomy.
Objective responses are however rare, and the mechanism is
unknown.

## Radiotherapy

This has a limited rôle in the palliation of symptoms from advanced local disease but an important rôle as a local treatment in the palliation of bone pain. In addition, widespread painful metastatic prostatic carcinoma refractory to hormonal manipulation is probably the best indication for palliative double hemi-body irradiation. Large single fractions are given to each half of the body, separated by a month or six weeks to allow marrow recovery in the irradiated half. Acute toxicity can be well controlled with steroids, intravenous fluids and sedation: patients need to spend one or two nights in hospital for each fraction. About 80 per cent of patients experience significant pain relief which can last for a year or more.

## Hormonal drugs

### *Oestrogens*

Efficacy is comparable with that of orchidectomy, but side effects are greater and include nausea, fluid retention, impotence and gynaecomastia. Most serious is the risk of potentially fatal venous and arterial thrombosis, and higher doses are particularly hazardous. Side effects from oestrogen therapy have been reported to cause 15 per cent of deaths during the first year of treatment. It should not be prescribed for the elderly, those who have undergone recent surgery, or those with a past history of thromboembolisms, cardiac failure or severe hypertension, and should be stopped before any major surgery.

Stilboestrol in a dosage of 1 mg tds is sufficient to reduce the serum testosterone to castrate levels. A dose of only 1 mg daily does not achieve this, but nevertheless may be clinically as effective, and probably carries a lower risk of cardiovascular morbidity. There is no evidence of benefit from giving oestrogen treatment, or any other hormone manipulation, before it is warranted by symptoms. Very few patients will benefit from oestrogens given on relapse following orchidectomy.

*LHRH agonists*

A 'medical orchidectomy' is now feasible with luteinising hormone releasing hormone (LHRH) agonists such as buserelin and goserelin. These drugs cause an initial surge of pituitary luteinising hormone (LH) and hence testosterone secretion, but this is followed by 'down-grading' of the LHRH receptors in the pituitary, a block in LH production and a cessation of testicular androgen production. The initial surge in testosterone production can very occasionally lead to serious sequelae from temporary tumour stimulation, such as spinal cord compression. Other patients may experience an exacerbation of pain. Such stimulation can be blocked by the prior administration of an anti-androgen, and LHRH agonists should never initially be administered alone.

Treatment with LHRH agonists is attractive because the risk of cardiovascular morbidity is much lower than with oestrogens. These drugs do, however, need to be given parenterally. There is a subcutaneous depot preparation of goserelin with a duration of action of one month, which is convenient and ensures compliance. Buserelin can initially be given subcutaneously, but subsequently requires intranasal administration.

*Anti-androgens*

Cyproterone and flutamide also carry a much lower risk of cardiovascular morbidity, but gynaecomastia is a common side effect, particularly with flutamide. In the short term they may be used to predict the response to orchidectomy, but longer-term treatment tends to be followed by a secondary increase in gonadotrophin and androgen secretion, requiring higher doses of the drug to neutralise the effect. Unlike the other manoeuvres, they are, however, capable of blocking adrenal androgen production. Objective responses are seen in a minority of patients who have relapsed following an initially successful hormonal manoeuvre, but 40–50 per cent of patients experience some subjective improvement.

The concept of 'total androgen blockade', using a combination of an LHRH analogue and a continued anti-androgen is under evaluation: it is possible that the consequent greater androgen suppression may improve on the efficacy of single modality treatment.

*Other drugs*

Aminoglutethimide blocks adrenal androgen and cortisol production, but can cause a rash and drowsiness; steroid replacement must be given simultaneously. It produces objective evidence of a response in about 20 per cent of patients who have relapsed following an initially successful hormonal manoeuvre, and some relief of pain in about 40 per cent, for a median duration of about six months.

Progestogens are also sometimes effective and may improve appetite and sense of well-being. The antifungal agent ketoconazole can inhibit adrenal and testicular androgen production in high dosage. These drugs are occasionally used as second-line therapy after failure of initial treatment, but unfortunately only a small minority of patients will derive significant benefit.

## Cytotoxic chemotherapy

Response rates to cytotoxic drugs are low and the duration of any responses short. Estramustine phosphate is a combination of the cytotoxic agent mustine and oestradiol. Response rates comparable to that with orchidectomy and pure oestrogens are seen when the drug is used on previously untreated patients. Significant efficacy has also been reported in the treatment of patients who have relapsed on first-line treatment. It is claimed that the oestradiol takes the mustine into the malignant cells, but the contribution of the mustine component to efficacy is uncertain.

## Follow-up

The outcome following radical treatment depends on the efficacy in achieving local control and the presence or absence of metastatic disease. Local failure cannot be salvaged and there can be no prospect of cure for metastatic disease, thus follow-up cannot improve the chance of ultimate cure, and management after initial treatment should be dictated by symptoms. However, patients with incidentally discovered impalpable and untreated carcinoma should be followed up in order to detect local tumour progression, which might warrant radical treatment.

The sequential estimation of prostatic acid phosphatase or other markers, such as the more sensitive prostate-specific antigen, can provide an objective indication of the response to treatment. It may allow earlier discontinuation of ineffective treatment, and earlier institution of alternative treatment, but it is not established that this is of any advantage compared with an expectant policy based on symptoms.

## Practice points

1 Supraclavicular fossa palpation, serum acid and alkaline phosphatase estimations and a chest X-ray are mandatory investigations prior to radical treatment. Isotope bone scans are often performed, but they pick up very few patients with metastatic bone disease in the absence of relevant symptoms or an elevated serum alkaline phosphatase.

2 There is no justification for routine follow-up bone scans in asymptomatic patients.

3 Weakness and limb aching is sometimes attributable to paraneoplastic hypophosphataemia. The abnormal biochemistry and symptoms usually respond well to 1 α-hydroxycholecalciferol (see Chapter 13 on metabolic disturbances).

**NOTES**

# NOTES

# CHAPTER 33

# Renal Carcinoma

The annual incidence is approximately six per 100,000 population and the male/female ratio 2:1. The great majority of malignant kidney tumours in adults are adenocarcinomas, sometimes called hypernephromas because it was once erroneously thought that they derived from adrenal tissue rather than the renal tubules. The cells are often large and contain clear cytoplasm, and these tumours are often referred to as 'clear cell' carcinomas. The majority of primary and metastatic tumours are very well vascularised, and this can be demonstrated by arteriography. About 5 per cent of renal carcinomas arise from the renal pelvis and are transitional cell carcinomas, deriving from the urothelium which extends from the renal pelvis to the bladder.

Overall about 30 per cent of patients are cured. The chance of cure is doubled if there is no renal capsule, nodal or renal vein involvement. The prognosis is worse for male patients, those with a high ESR, and those with adenocarcinomas of other than 'clear cell' histology.

Metastases occasionally occur many years after nephrectomy for adenocarcinoma and can be truly solitary. Spontaneous regression of metastases following removal of the primary adenocarcinoma is well recognised but very rare.

## Risk factors

Smoking; long-term phenacetin; possibly polycystic kidneys.

## Spread

This occurs locally through the renal capsule and to distant sites by both lymphatic (para-aortic nodes) and venous routes. Renal vein involvement is quite common. Haematogenous spread occurs especially to lungs, liver and bones.

## Symptoms and signs

Haematuria
Abdominal mass
Pain
Weight loss
Fever
Anaemia

# Treatment

## Radical

### Surgery

Nephrectomy is essential for cure. The value of more radical procedures involving removal of peri-renal fat, retro-renal fascia and regional lymph nodes is unproven. Excision of a solitary metastasis from an adenocarcinoma can be followed by prolonged survival and is sometimes curative, especially when the metastasis becomes apparent several years after nephrectomy. Excision of the primary tumour in the presence of metastases, in the hope of subsequent spontaneous regression, is not justified unless required for local symptom control. The remote chance of benefit is substantially outweighed by the morbidity and risk of death from surgery.

### Radiotherapy

Pre- or post-operative radiotherapy to the renal bed and nearby lymph nodes has been claimed to improve survival but is of unproven value.

## Palliative

### Surgery

Nephrectomy can be valuable for pain and haematuria. Renal artery embolisation can provide useful palliation with less morbidity than nephrectomy, although pain, fever and hypertension may occur immediately afterwards.

### Radiotherapy

Pain and haematuria from the primary tumour can be improved by radiotherapy. It is also usually effective in relieving metastatic bone pain.

### Cytotoxic chemotherapy

This has very little efficacy.

### Hormone therapy

Progestogens (e.g. medroxyprogesterone acetate 400 mg daily) are occasionally of benefit for patients with adenocarcinoma, but objective responses are seen in <10 per cent of patients. Other patients may experience some improvement in appetite and sense of well-being, due to the non-specific steroidal effect. The side effects of progestogens however include thrombophlebitis, diabetes and hypercalcaemia, and routine use is probably not justified.

### Interferon

Responses are seen in about 25 per cent of patients with adenocarcinoma, but these are usually partial and last only about six months. Troublesome toxicity is common, particularly 'flu-like' symptoms.

## Follow-up

For almost all patients the long-term outcome is determined at presentation or by the completion of treatment. However, six-monthly chest radiography for ten years may be justified in order to detect a solitary metastasis at an early stage.

Multifocal urothelial malignancy occurs in about 30 per cent of patients with transitional cell carcinoma. Follow-up with urine cytology and cystoscopy is justified after radical treatment to detect further tumours on the other side and in the bladder.

## Practice points

1 Overt metastatic disease must be excluded prior to radical treatment. Supraclavicular fossae examination and chest radiography are essential.
2 Varicocoele may indicate left renal vein involvement.
3 Lower limb oedema may indicate involvement of inferior vena cava or para-aortic lymph nodes.
4 Hypercalcaemia may occur due to humoral factor(s) secreted by the primary tumour and does not necessarily indicate bone metastases.
5 Reversible hepatosplenomegaly and abnormal liver function tests occur in about 10 per cent of patients, and are also attributable to a humoral mechanism.
6 About 25 per cent of patients have hypertension associated with raised serum renin levels.

**NOTES**

# NOTES

# Sarcomas

# CHAPTER 34

# Sarcomas

The total annual incidence of sarcomatous tumours is approximately three per 100,000 population. These are malignant neoplasms of mesodermal origin and can arise almost anywhere. The more common varieties are osteosarcoma, Ewing's sarcoma (arising in bone but possibly of a pluripotent mesenchymal origin), chondrosarcoma, fibrosarcoma and 'malignant fibrous histiocytoma', rhabdomyosarcoma and liposarcoma. Osteosarcoma, Ewing's sarcoma and rhabdomyosarcoma have a particular predilection to occur in childhood or adolescence.

These tumours often develop in the limbs and, apart from primary skin carcinomas, are the only malignant tumours that do so. However, the bones and connective tissues of the trunk are also quite often involved and leiomyosarcomas characteristically arise from the smooth muscle of the gastrointestinal tract. Kaposi's sarcoma is a tumour of endothelial origin that is now much more common with the advent of AIDS. It is usually more aggressive in AIDS patients and may extensively involve not only the skin but also the hard palate, gut and other viscera.

These tumours vary enormously in their malignant potential. At one end of the spectrum are extremely indolent neoplasms (quite often liposarcomas) which seem hardly to grow at all. They show no evidence of metastatic potential, exhibit very infrequent mitoses on histological examination and may be very difficult to distinguish from benign neoplasms. At the other end of the spectrum are rapidly growing tumours which metastasise widely. Unfortunately more neoplasms are nearer the latter end than the former. The substantial majority of patients with osteosarcoma and Ewing's sarcoma have microscopic distant metastases at presentation. Overall probably not more than one-third of patients are cured.

## Risk factors

Ionising radiation; neurofibromatosis (fibrosarcoma); lymphoedema (angiosarcoma); AIDS and other causes of immunosuppression (Kaposi's sarcoma); Paget's disease (osteosarcoma); vinyl chloride (hepatic angiosarcoma).

## Spread

Local invasion and blood-borne dissemination are the commonest forms of spread. Lung metastases are very common. Lymphatic spread does occur but is relatively uncommon. Spread through tissue planes is a characteristic feature of soft tissue sarcomas; these tumours sometimes form a 'pseudo-capsule' by compression of the surrounding tissue but this is not a true capsule and it always contains cancerous elements.

## Symptoms and signs

Soft tissue or bony mass
Pain (particularly osteosarcoma)
Violaceous initially flat then raised skin and mucous membrane nodule(s) (Kaposi's sarcoma)
Local and systemic features suggestive of infection (Ewing's sarcoma)

# Treatment

## Radical

### Surgery

This is the mainstay of treatment for apparently localised sarcomas. Complete excision with a good resection margin is the surest way of achieving local control. For limb lesions this has traditionally involved amputation for many tumours, particularly osteosarcomas. An adequate margin has most commonly required transection one joint above the tumour-bearing bone, necessitating fore or hind quarter amputations for some patients. However, modern prosthetic implant techniques can now avoid amputation for some patients with bone cancer, without adversely affecting survival.

For patients with soft tissue sarcomas lesser operations than amputation have proved feasible in about half of those with primary limb tumours, but the surgical technique is crucial to success at any site. Mere local excision with little or no margin of normal tissue carries an approximately 75 per cent chance of local recurrence: optimal surgery involves careful preoperative planning followed by a radical operation involving removal of the entire anatomical compartment where this is feasible. The biopsy site should be included in the specimen and ideally the tumour should not be seen during the procedure. Such surgery is however quite often not feasible, even in the most experienced hands, due to the size or extent of the tumour.

It has become recognised that limb-sparing procedures and other more conservative operations are acceptable for some patients. The advent of effective cytotoxic chemotherapy for osteosarcoma has facilitated non-amputational surgery for some patients, involving removal of the involved bone and prosthetic replacement. For soft tissue sarcomas, where radical surgery is not possible, or would inevitably involve amputation, it has been demonstrated that more conservative surgery followed by radical radiotherapy to the anatomical compartment can achieve an equivalent rate of local control.

Surgical resection of pulmonary metastases, even when multiple, should be considered for patients with osteosarcoma, and also for some with soft tissue sarcomas. The existence of effective cytotoxic chemotherapy for osteosarcoma (which can eliminate micrometastases) makes surgical treatment for lung metastases a particularly appealing option for many patients with this tumour, even if metastases are present at the outset. Comparable efficacy is not found with cytotoxic chemotherapy for soft-tissue sarcomas. For metastases presenting after primary treatment the length of the intervening disease-free interval seems to correlate with the chance of benefit from resection. For patients with osteosarcoma, resection of lung metastases can contribute substantially to long-term survival, and almost certainly to the chance of cure.

## Radiotherapy

The majority of sarcomas are bulky and relatively radioresistant. Ewing's sarcomas, in contrast, are usually very radiosensitive and for these radiotherapy and not surgery is often the local treatment of choice. For other sarcomas radiation now has very little place as a single modality in radical treatment, but high doses can eradicate microscopic disease residual after surgery. Radical radiotherapy has a particularly important rôle in achieving local control after less than radical surgery for soft tissue sarcomas. Nevertheless, effective doses have a high propensity to cause quite marked fibrosis, particularly in the limbs, and this can substantially impair function and can cause pain. As with surgery careful attention to technique is essential: part of the cross-sectional area of the limb must be excluded from the treatment volume in order to avoid severe lymphoedema.

Adjuvant low-dose irradiation to both lungs has been advocated for osteosarcoma. Although one study has shown comparable efficacy to cytotoxic chemotherapy there is currently little enthusiasm for this approach in routine practice.

## Cytotoxic chemotherapy

This has no place in radical treatment as a single modality, and is not effective as an adjuvant treatment for other than osteosarcomas and Ewing's sarcoma. Adjuvant chemotherapy improves survival in osteosarcoma and Ewing's sarcoma and probably also improves the chance of cure. Most osteosarcoma regimens involve the use of high-dose methotrexate and leucovorin rescue together with other drugs including adriamycin, actinomycin D, cisplatin, bleomycin and cyclophosphamide. In some centres a combination of drugs is given pre-operatively, with continuation post-operatively with either the same or another combination depending on the initial response.

**Palliative**

Surgery

This has little use as a treatment of purely palliative intent, but amputation may substantially improve the quality of life for some patients with uncontrolled primary tumours in the presence of incurable metastases.

Radiotherapy

This, too, is of little purely palliative value since most tumours require rather high doses for a significant response. An exception is superficial Kaposi's sarcoma in AIDS patients, where excellent palliation may be achieved with very short courses of superficial radiotherapy.

Cytotoxic chemotherapy

This is usually given with radical intent for osteosarcoma but many will derive only palliative benefit. Response rates are considerably lower for soft tissue sarcomas and extremely low for chondrosarcoma. About one-third of patients with soft tissue sarcomas respond to single agent ifosfamide for on average about nine months. About 30 per cent of AIDS patients with Kaposi's sarcoma show some response to cytotoxic chemotherapy, but these are usually of short duration. Such marrow and immuno-suppressive treatment is fraught with problems in this group of patients.

Interferon

Alpha-interferon produces useful responses in about 40 per cent of AIDS patients with Kaposi's sarcoma who have not previously experienced opportunistic infections. In patients who have had opportunistic infections the response rates are much lower.

**Follow-up**

Close follow-up with regular chest radiology (including CT scans) is reasonable for most patients with osteosarcoma, since the discovery of local recurrence in conservatively treated limbs (or any other excisable local recurrence) or lung metastases may lead to further useful, and potentially curable, treatment. A similar policy but with conventional chest radiographs rather than CT scans is probably justifiable for the majority of patients treated for soft tissue sarcoma, with the addition of CT scans wherever a local recurrence might be amenable to further surgery.

## Practice points

1 Patients with apparently localised disease and other than very low-grade neoplasms should usually have CT scans of the chest and primary site in their initial assessment. The discovery of lung metastases may usefully influence management in either a more aggressive or conservative direction, depending on the histology, site and extent of the primary tumour.
2 Aspiration cytology is usually not acceptable for diagnosis. A trephine, tru-cut, or often an incisional biopsy is required, choosing a carefully placed route which will not compromise subsequent surgery.
3 Local treatment with limb-sparing surgery with or without radiotherapy should be carefully planned beforehand, with meticulous attention to both surgical and radiotherapeutic technique. The mere 'shelling out' of soft tissue sarcomas is hardly ever curative. Arteriography can be very helpful in planning sophisticated surgery.
4 Baseline CT scans of the primary site after the completion of local treatment with surgery with or without radiotherapy are often of value in the assessment of subsequent scans arranged at follow-up. Liposarcomas, because of their fatty content, usually show up very well on CT scans.

# NOTES

# CHAPTER 35

# Skin Cancer

The documented annual incidence is approximately 50 per 100,000 population but the true incidence is almost certainly higher because there is under-reporting. The great majority of skin cancers are basal cell carcinomas (rodent ulcers). These almost never metastasise and the cure rate is virtually 100 per cent. The next most common type is squamous carcinoma. These can metastasise but the cure rate is about 95 per cent. Most basal and squamous carcinomas arise on the face, ears, scalp and back.

There are about six per 100,000 cases annually of malignant melanoma. They occur on any part of the body and can arise on mucous membranes. These are far more serious tumours with a cure rate of only 50–60 per cent. The outlook is slightly better for females. The chance of cure with melanomas <1 mm thick is >90 per cent, but the risk of death rises rapidly with increasing thickness.

Other skin malignancies include Bowen's disease (squamous carcinoma-in-situ); mycosis fungoides, a T-cell lymphoma which initially is confined to the skin but then tends to spread to lymph nodes and eventually to the viscera; and B-cell lymphomas. The lymphomas are highly radiosensitive. Solar or actinic keratoses are very common and occasionally progress to squamous carcinoma.

## Basal and Squamous Carcinomas

### Risk factors

Ultraviolet irradiation and fair skin; scars; immunosuppression; albinism; arsenic; topical coal tar and benzpyrene.

## Spread

Basal cell carcinomas invade only locally. Squamous carcinomas spread to regional lymph nodes, but blood-borne spread is extremely rare.

## Treatment

### Surgery

Complete excision is the surest treatment for any skin neoplasm. It is also often the quickest and best-tolerated approach. However, surgery on the face is sometimes more complex, involving more sophisticated plastic surgical techniques to achieve adequate cosmesis. Surgery is the treatment of choice for basal or squamous carcinomas arising on the trunk or limbs, and for lymphadenopathy. Other minor surgical techniques such as curettage and cryosurgery can achieve eradication of the majority of basal cell carcinomas, but are quite often followed by recurrence.

### Radiotherapy

Superficial treatment is highly effective for basal and squamous carcinomas arising on the head and neck and the cosmetic result is usually good. It is somewhat better for more protracted regimens, e.g. 10–15 daily fractions, but much shorter and sharper courses are often acceptable. Longer courses are, however, essential for lesions on the pinna, to reduce the risk of cartilaginous necrosis. Radiotherapy is poorly tolerated on the trunk and limbs; healing is slow and there is an appreciable incidence of long-term necrosis, particularly on the extremities.

### Cytotoxic chemotherapy

Topical 5-fluorouracil is an effective treatment for solar keratoses, Bowen's disease, and very superficial basal cell carcinomas.

## Follow-up

Fairly close follow-up is justified for most patients after treatment for squamous carcinoma. This is to detect local or lymph node recurrence at an early stage. A reasonable schedule would be two-monthly initially, increasing after a year to three- to four-monthly and further after two years, discontinuing at five years. Patients with basal cell carcinomas do not usually require prolonged follow-up.

It should be noted that patients with basal or squamous carcinomas should be warned that they are at risk of further malignancies and advised to avoid excessive sun exposure, to wear hats in the sun, to use barrier creams and report any new lesions promptly.

# Malignant Melanoma

### Risk factors

Ultraviolet irradiation and fair skin; tendency to burn easily and tan poorly when exposed to sunlight; multiple naevi and heavy freckling (including familial melanocytic naevi syndrome).

### Spread

Melanomas spread both via lymphatics to nearby skin and regional lymph nodes, and via the blood stream. The chance of distant spread from melanoma is closely related to the thickness of the primary growth. It increases markedly once the thickness is over 1 mm and distant metastases will be present in about 75 per cent of those over 4 mm.

### Symptoms and signs

New enlarging pigmented lesion
Enlargement of pre-existing mole, particularly with:
    Irregular border
    Irregular surface
    Heterogeneity of pigmentation
    Itching
    Bleeding

Satellite lesions
Multiple widespread new cutaneous or sub-cutaneous nodules
Lymphadenopathy
Hepatomegaly

## Treatment – radical

### Surgery

It is always the treatment of choice for primary melanoma, where a good margin is important to prevent local recurrence: where feasible this should be 2 cm for lesions under 1 mm thickness and 3–5 cm for thicker lesions, with skin grafting.

There is some evidence to suggest that elective regional lymph node dissection improves the chance of cure for patients with intermediate thickness melanomas (1.5–3.5 mm). It is probably not effective for those with thinner lesions because of their low incidence of spread, and neither for those with thicker lesions because most will have widespread dissemination.

There is no evidence that incisional biopsy of malignant melanoma adversely affects prognosis, but excisional biopsy is preferable whenever possible because malignant change may not have occurred throughout a previously benign lesion, and full information on thickness enables better planning of any further surgery to the primary or to lymph nodes.

### Radiotherapy

Melanoma is usually a radioresistant tumour and radiotherapy has little rôle in radical treatment.

### Cytotoxic chemotherapy

This has been given adjuvantly after surgery for apparently localised disease, intravenously and via arterial limb perfusion, but there is as yet no evidence that it improves the chance of cure.

**Treatment – palliative**

Surgery

Resection of troublesome soft tissue melanoma metastases, where feasible, can be the best tolerated as well as the quickest way of achieving palliation.

Radiotherapy

This is sometimes given with palliative intent for patients with advanced melanoma. The results are generally rather disappointing but gratifying responses are sometimes seen. There is some evidence to suggest that regimens involving larger dose fractions may be more effective.

Cytotoxic chemotherapy

Drugs with some efficacy in advanced melanoma include vindesine, DTIC and the nitrosoureas. However the response rates are usually only about 25 per cent (a little higher for some toxic combinations) and the duration of response is usually only a few months.

Immunotherapy

Spontaneous regression occasionally occurs in patients with melanoma, and individual deposits in patients with multiple lesions quite frequently show minor fluctuations in size. These observations have engendered some enthusiasm for immunological approaches.

Injection of BCG into melanoma lesions results in local regression in about two-thirds of patients. In a small percentage there is regression in uninjected nodules, but usually only in those near to the injection site. Complete responses are occasionally seen.

Alpha interferon produces responses in about 20 per cent of patients, lasting on average four to six months.

**Follow-up**

Fairly close follow-up is appropriate for most patients after surgery for melanoma, with a schedule similar to that suggested above for squamous carcinoma. This is primarily in order to be able to offer early surgery for regional lymph node metastases.

Patients should be warned that they are at risk of further malignancy, and advised to avoid excessive sun exposure, to wear hats in the sun, to use barrier creams and report any new lesions or changes in moles promptly.

**NOTES**

# CHAPTER 36

# Stomach Carcinoma

The incidence is approximately 20 per 100,000 population annually and the male/female ratio 3:2. The incidence is declining in the western world. Adenocarcinomas constitute 95 per cent of the total. Most tumours are ulcerative and develop in the lower third of the stomach and rarely arise from the greater curvature. They very frequently extend some way beyond what is macroscopically apparent and thus most tumours present at an advanced stage; there is histological evidence of regional lymph node involvement in approximately 50 per cent. The only chance of cure is with surgery but overall approximately 20 per cent survive one year and only about 5 per cent are cured. However, patients found to have localised disease at operation have an approximately 25 per cent chance of cure.

### Risk factors

Family history; pernicious anaemia; surgery for benign peptic ulcer; villous adenoma; possibly blood group A, intestinal metaplasia, asbestos, smoked and salted foods, milk from bracken-eating cows.

### Spread

Diffuse local submucosal infiltration; regional lymph nodes; liver; trans-coelomic.

323

## Symptoms and signs

Symptoms are often vague and non-specific
Weight loss
Epigastric pain
Anorexia
Nausea/vomiting
Haematemesis
Palpable upper abdominal tumour (indicates incurability)
Supraclavicular lymphadenopathy

# Treatment

## Radical

### Surgery

Resection offers the only chance of cure. Approximately 75 per cent of patients are initially considered operable, and approximately 50 per cent undergo resection. The remainder are discovered to be inoperable on opening the abdomen. The procedures used include sub-total gastrectomy, total gastrectomy, and extended total gastrectomy in which the body and tail of the pancreas are also removed. Regional lymph nodes, omentum, and often the spleen are removed, and continuity with the duodenum or jejunum re-established by a variety of reconstructive procedures. Operative mortality is usually approximately 10 per cent.

### Combined modality

Radiotherapy to this region is not well tolerated. However, it has been used before surgery in an attempt to improve resectability, after surgery for residual disease, and also intra-operatively when a single very localised high dose can be given to the tumour bed. Evidence of benefit has so far been scanty and there is no justification for the routine use of radiotherapy. A variety of regimens of adjuvant cytotoxic chemotherapy has been investigated but there is no good evidence that this approach either is of benefit.

## Palliative

### Surgery

Both sub-total gastrectomy and bypass procedures may sometimes be justified in an attempt to palliate incurable disease.

### Radiotherapy and cytotoxic chemotherapy

These have been tried singly and in combination but the results have not been particularly encouraging. Approximately 30 per cent of selected patients may respond to the most effective drug combinations, and the responses may last on average about nine months, but the side-effects militate against chemotherapy being considered for more than a carefully selected minority.

## Follow-up

There is little justification for close oncological follow-up after radical surgery since clinical 'recurrence' is inevitably fatal and only symptomatic management is appropriate. However, there is enthusiasm in a few centres for 'second look' operations for patients who appear to be free from disease following primary treatment, with the aim of removing any discovered local 'recurrence' when it is still operable.

## Practice points

1 Overt metastatic disease must be excluded prior to planned radical surgery. Supraclavicular fossae examination, chest radiography and liver function tests are essential and CT scanning of the upper abdomen highly advisable.
2 Post-gastrectomy complications include the dumping syndrome, stomal ulcer, blind loop syndrome with malabsorption, vitamin B12 deficiency due to lack of intrinsic factor, and recrudescence of pulmonary tuberculosis. Patients must be given vitamin B12.

# NOTES

# CHAPTER 37

# Testicular Germ Cell Tumours

Testicular cancer is the commonest malignancy in men under the age of 35 years: the annual incidence is approximately four new cases per 100,000 males. The great majority of malignant testicular tumours are tumours of the germ cell epithelium lining the testicular tubules, and are either teratomas or seminomas or combinations of the two. Seminomas tend to occur in a slightly older (more middle-aged) population. Seminomas are very commonly confined to the testis but metastases are present in about half of all patients with teratoma.

Germ cell tumours very occasionally arise at other sites (such as the mediastinum) due to the presence of germ cell 'rests' left behind during embryonal gonadal descent but metastases from primary testicular tumours are sometimes wrongly interpreted as being extra gonadal primaries. Diagnosis of these can be made only after negative testicular biopsies, and even these are not conclusive since a small primary tumour can be missed.

Seminoma cells look much like those normally lining the germinal epithelium. In teratomas the pluripotential nature of these germ cells becomes apparent because differentiation takes place to somatic tissues (endo-, meso- or ectoderm) and/or extraembryonic tissues (trophoblast or yolk sac). There is great variation amongst teratomas according to the varying representation of these different elements, and the degree of differentiation and malignancy. However, unlike ovarian teratomas no male teratoma can be considered benign; even very differentiated teratomas consisting of apparently mature tissues can metastasise.

Malignant non-invading cells (carcinoma in-situ) are often seen in tubules adjacent to malignant tumours and this change is found in about 5 per cent of biopsies taken from the otherwise apparently normal contralateral testis, rising to about 25 per cent if there is a history of cryptorchidism or atrophy. Probably about 50 per cent of carcinomas in-situ become invasive within five years; overall about 2 per cent of patients develop contralateral invasive tumours but this figure is probably reduced by chemotherapy, and by radiotherapy if the scrotum is included in the treatment volume.

Normal yolk sac produces alpha-fetoprotein (AFP) and normal trophoblast produces beta human chorionic gonadotrophin (β-HCG). The majority of testicular teratomas produce sufficient quantities of one or other, or both, of these hormones to result in detectable raised serum levels. A small percentage of seminomas produce raised β-HCG levels but they do not produce raised AFP concentrations. About 50 per cent of seminomas produce raised placental alkaline phosphatase levels and both teratomas and seminomas often cause raised lactate dehydrogenase (LDH) levels. The presence of these raised 'markers' enables much more sensitive monitoring than is possible with clinical examination and radiography. The production of human chorionic somatomammotrophin by some teratomas explains the occurrence of gynaecomastia in some patients.

The natural history of some 'mature' teratomas can be extremely long, extending over decades, but for most germ cell tumours late recurrence is unusual; the great majority of 'recurrences' will occur within two years after treatment. An interesting phenomenon is the persistence of masses of metastatic tumour after chemotherapy, which would appear to have been successful as judged by the marker response. Histological examination reveals that in one-third of such patients the tissue is necrotic, in another third there is obvious persistent malignancy, and in the other third there has been differentiation to mature well-differentiated (but still malignant) teratoma, which may subsequently give rise to other malignancies, e.g. sarcoma.

There has been a dramatic improvement in the outlook for patients with advanced disease during the past fifteen years, with the advent of cisplatinum-containing cytotoxic chemotherapy. Even patients with very extensive metastatic disease can now expect a 75 per cent chance of complete remission, and about 75 per cent of these will be cured. Overall about 85 per cent of patients with teratoma and 95 per cent with seminoma can now be cured. The chance of metastatic disease is increased when there is lymphatic or blood vessel invasion in the primary tumour, and when it is undifferentiated. The prognosis is also worse with large tumour bulk, particularly multiple large lung metastases, very high serum marker levels (AFP >500 KU/l or β-HCG >1000 IU/l), liver, bone or brain metastases, choriocarcinoma and gynaecomastia.

### Risk factors

Undescended testis; gonadal dysgenesis; probably torsion of the testis; possibly maternal oestrogen ingestion and obesity during pregnancy, and industrial exposure to dimethylformide (e.g. leather tanners). Orchidopexy does not reduce risk.

### Spread

The dense fibrous tunica albuginea covering the testis substantially restricts local spread, but this can occur along the spermatic cord. Distant spread occurs via lymphatics to the para-aortic nodes and higher, and via the blood stream to lungs, brain and other organs. Providing the tunica albuginea is not breached by surgery (including past orchidopexy) or tumour invasion there is an exceedingly low risk of lymphatic spread to the groin. About 15 per cent and 30 per cent respectively, of patients with clinically localised seminoma and teratoma, have occult metastases, but these figures are higher in patients with invasion of testicular lymphatics or veins, and in patients with teratomas showing undifferentiated tumour or no evidence of a yolk sac component.

### Symptoms and signs

Testicular mass, painless or painful. Often injury draws attention to it.

Mass is OFTEN thought to be, and treated as, orchitis
Back pain (para-aortic nodes)
Gynaecomastia
Supraclavicular lymphadenopathy
Cough
Dyspnoea
Chest pain
Leg and genital oedema

# Treatment

## Radical

### Surgery

It is essential that serum should be sent for tumour marker estimation prior to surgery. This is in order to establish whether the particular tumour is producing markers and therefore how useful subsequent estimations will be in determining whether there is residual disease after surgery, in follow-up after apparently successful surgery and in monitoring the response to chemotherapy.

Orchidectomy must always be performed via an inguinal incision: a scrotal incision may allow malignant cells to implant in the scrotum and then spread to inguinal lymph nodes. If possible spermatic vein blood should be sent for marker estimation as concentrations will be higher than in blood elsewhere.

Residual masses of metastatic teratoma after effective chemotherapy should be monitored for a few months by plain films or CT scans as necessary, and if persistent they should be removed when possible. Retroperitoneal lymphadenectomy is a difficult operation which in the United Kingdom is usually undertaken as a potentially curative procedure for residual para-aortic tumour after chemotherapy. Elsewhere, particularly in the United States, radical lymphadenectomy is often undertaken as a staging and potentially therapeutic procedure as part of initial management. Loss of ejaculation is very common after this operation, but some patients develop retrograde ejaculation which can be successfully treated with imipramine. Resection of residual metastatic lung tumour after chemotherapy is also undertaken with curative intent.

## Radiotherapy

Seminomas are extremely radio-sensitive and it has been common practice to irradiate routinely the para-aortic lymph nodes (±pelvic nodes) even when the tumour appears to have been localised to the testis, because well-tolerated low doses will eradicate microscopic metastases. Teratomas are less radiosensitive and respond so well to modern chemotherapy that radiotherapy does not now play much part in their management. There is accumulating evidence that platinum-containing chemotherapy is as effective for seminoma as it is for teratoma, and the role of radiotherapy, at least in the treatment of extensive or bulky metastatic disease, is declining. Formerly radiotherapy was offered for mediastinal or lung spread but had low curative potential. The existence of effective chemotherapy for seminoma is encouraging policies of close follow-up rather than routine adjuvant radiotherapy. Radiotherapy should not now be given as initial treatment for patients with any advanced testicular tumour, since it reduces bone marrow tolerance to chemotherapy.

Low dose radiotherapy appears to be a successful treatment, at least in the short term, for carcinoma in-situ.

## Cytotoxic chemotherapy

For the treatment of teratomas, cisplatin needs to be given in conjunction with other cytotoxic drugs such as bleomycin, etoposide and vinblastine. Chemotherapy is indicated for advanced disease and also for patients with apparently localised tumour but poor prognostic factors. Treatment is toxic and is given on an in-patient basis with intravenous hydration. Usually about four courses are given at monthly intervals. More aggressive disease may require the use of more intensive regimens, which may involve the addition of other drugs, before disease control can be achieved. An analogue of cisplatin, carboplatin, is substantially less toxic but it is not yet fully established that it has equal efficacy; however there have been encouraging reports of its efficacy as a single agent for advanced seminoma.

Renal function needs to be monitored closely. Other side effects of chemotherapy include severe nausea and vomiting, ototoxicity, skin pigmentation, Raynaud's phenomenon, peripheral neuropathy and lung fibrosis. Azoospermia is inevitable in almost all patients but about 50 per cent recover normal spermatogenesis two to three years after chemotherapy. All patients should be offered sperm storage prior to chemotherapy. There is no evidence for an increased incidence of abnormal offspring to fathers (or mothers) who received chemotherapy prior to conception.

## Follow-up

Patients who relapse after surgery alone can be salvaged by chemotherapy, and patients who relapse after chemotherapy can be salvaged by further surgery or further chemotherapy. It seems probable that the chance of success of salvage treatment is increased if relapse is detected at an early stage. Thus close follow-up is justified, particularly during the first two years. Follow-up investigations include regular tumour marker estimations, chest X-rays and CT scans of chest and abdomen. Particularly close follow-up is required for patients with apparently localised tumours treated with orchidectomy alone.

## Practice points

1   Delayed diagnosis is still common. Many patients are thought to have orchitis or an orthopaedic cause for back pain.
2   Scrotal ultrasound is helpful pre-operatively if there is any doubt about the diagnosis. It may prevent a scrotal incision for supposed benign pathology.
3   Serum for AFP and β-HCG must be sent prior to orchidectomy (and spermatic vein blood at operation).
4   Orchidectomy must be performed via an inguinal incision.
5   Biopsy of the contralateral testis should be considered, especially for patients with a history of maldescent or sub-fertility.

6 Patients should usually be offered sperm storage prior to cytotoxic chemotherapy or pelvic radiotherapy, but this must not be allowed to delay significantly treatment for aggressive disease. Many patients are already sub-fertile.

7 Respiratory distress syndrome can follow cytotoxic chemotherapy for extensive lung metastases: treatment should be given initially in reduced dosage with steroid cover.

8 Transient gynaecomastia is a common occurrence after the completion of chemotherapy but carries no prognostic significance.

9 Patients should be encouraged to undertake regular self-palpation of the remaining testis.

## NOTES

# CHAPTER 38

# Thyroid Cancer

The annual incidence is approximately two per 100,000 population. It is over twice as common in females than males. About 90 per cent of thyroid cancers arise from the follicular epithelium and some of these can look remarkably like normal thyroid. Well-differentiated follicular carcinomas may exhibit almost normal-looking follicles containing colloid; less differentiated tumours have a more solid component. Papillary carcinomas are often well differentiated but contain papilliferous epithelial processes and also often contain colloid. Many tumours contain mixed papillary and follicular elements, in which case they are classified as papillary carcinomas.

Differentiated thyroid carcinomas, both follicular and papillary, but particularly the former, may retain the normal gland's ability to take up iodine, and also some responsiveness to normal endocrine control (TSH). Papillary carcinomas are usually indolent tumours, even though they quite commonly spread to neck nodes. Follicular carcinomas are usually more aggressive, with a greater tendency to invade blood vessels and disseminate widely. Anaplastic carcinomas are highly undifferentiated tumours which grow and infiltrate rapidly. All these carcinomas have a tendency towards multifocal (quite often bilateral) involvement. Papillary carcinomas constitute about 60 per cent of the total, follicular 15 per cent and anaplastic 15 per cent. Differentiated carcinomas are found in up to 5 per cent of people dying of other diseases.

The remaining 10 per cent of thyroid cancers are non-follicular malignancies: medullary carcinomas, which arise from the parafollicular C-cells which normally produce calcitonin, and lymphomas. Medullary carcinomas produce calcitonin and many other humoral agents, including prostaglandins and vaso-active intestinal polypeptide. About 80 per cent of patients with papillary carcinoma and 60 per cent with follicular and medullary carcinoma are cured. Anaplastic carcinomas carry a very poor prognosis: the chance of cure is less than 10 per cent.

### Risk factors

Ionising radiation, particularly in children, but not radio-iodine for thyrotoxicosis; family history (20 per cent of those with medullary carcinoma).

### Spread

Local infiltration through the capsule; lymphatic to neck nodes; blood-borne to lungs and bones particularly.

### Symptoms and signs

Hard thyroid nodule
Neck lymphadenopathy
Watery diarrhoea (30 per cent with medullary carcinoma)

# Treatment

### Radical

#### Surgery

This is the initial treatment of choice for all operable carcinomas. It is most unusual for a thyroidectomy to be truly total: even when every attempt has been made to remove all the gland there is nearly always some remaining. However, the more aggressive the surgery the higher the risk of hypoparathyroidism and vocal cord palsy due to damage to recurrent laryngeal nerves. Damage to the external laryngeal nerves is quite common, causing post-operative voice changes, such as huskiness and poor volume, in a significant minority of patients.

A 'total' or near total thyroidectomy is undoubtedly the treatment of choice for medullary carcinoma. It is favoured by some for follicular and papillary carcinomas, although others favour a sub-total thyroidectomy (removal of the involved lobe, isthmus and most of the opposite lobe); the minimal acceptable operation is a total lobectomy. Radio-iodine ablation (see below) is easier if more thyroid tissue has been removed.

There is substantial controversy concerning the treatment of differentiated thyroid cancers, particularly papillary carcinomas. Their usually indolent nature had been seen as a justification for conservative treatment with thyroid lobectomy alone. Their propensity for multifocal involvement and the ability of many growths to take up cancerocidal doses of radio-iodine have however been used to justify 'total' or 'near total' thyroidectomy followed by radio-iodine. These contrasting philosophies have not been compared in a prospective randomised study.

Surgery is quite often required for neck lymphadenopathy. Prophylactic neck dissection is not now usually recommended except for some patients with medullary carcinoma. For patients with papillary and follicular carcinomas local excision of involved lymph glands is usually adequate.

## External radiotherapy

External radiotherapy is only occasionally given for differentiated carcinomas, but can be justified (perhaps in conjunction with radio-iodine) when there is known residual local disease after surgery for advanced tumours. Many anaplastic carcinomas are inoperable at presentation and then external radiotherapy holds the only (very slim) chance of cure. External radiotherapy is usually the treatment of choice for patients with localised thyroid lymphoma.

## Radio-iodine

Differentiated carcinomas that show colloid formation may be capable of taking up cancerocidal doses of orally administered radio-iodine. High doses of radio-iodine are thus often administered to patients with follicular and papillary carcinomas (particularly the former). Radio-iodine is given at approximately three-monthly intervals, until scans show no residual isotope uptake in the neck or abnormally elsewhere. Some patients require only one or two doses, others rather more.

Even very well-differentiated carcinomas are almost always much less avid for iodine than normal thyroid and thus if there is residual normal thyroid tissue present most of the radio-iodine will be concentrated in the normal thyroid, and not usefully within any residual malignant tissue (locally or at metastatic sites). Complete ablation of the normal thyroid is therefore necessary before a cancerocidal effect is likely. Complete ablation is much more quickly achieved with radio-iodine if there is only very little thyroid remaining after surgery. It is usually hoped that the ablative dose given when scans subsequently show no residual uptake in the neck will destroy residual microscopic carcinoma in the neck or at metastatic sites. Radio-iodine is also given to patients with proven metastatic disease. When this is not particularly bulky there is a reasonable chance of cure even for those with widely disseminated disease.

Radio-iodine is usually very well tolerated, although if there is a substantial residue of normal thyroid at the time of the first administration the radiation uptake in the neck may be sufficient to cause some soreness and swelling. Very occasionally there is precipitation of acute thyrotoxicosis due to release of large amounts of thyroxine. Other occasional side effects include salivary gland swelling and soreness, nausea and vomiting, and amenorrhoea. Very rarely marrow suppression is seen with high cumulative doses and pulmonary radiation fibrosis in patients with lung metastases.

There is no place for radio-iodine in the management of other than follicular or papillary carcinomas.

## Thyroid replacement

Thyroid hormone replacement is essential for virtually all patients. However, for those with follicular or papillary carcinomas the replacement dose should be sufficient to suppress the plasma TSH concentration to just below the normal range, without causing overt thyrotoxicosis. This reduces endogenous TSH stimulation of any residual tumour. Either

T4 (e.g. 0.3 mg/day) or T3 (e.g. 20 µg tds) can be used but the latter is preferable when radio-iodine ablation is still proceeding.

Discontinuation of thyroid replacement is essential prior to the administration of radio-iodine, otherwise its uptake will be suppressed. Tri-iodothyronine (T3) has a shorter half-life than thyroxine (T4) and can be discontinued only one week to ten days before radio-iodine administration, compared with a month for T4. Sometimes additional TSH is administered to stimulate isotope uptake further.

### Cytotoxic chemotherapy

This is indicated only for lymphomas.

## Palliative

### Surgery

This has very little place in palliative management.

### Radiotherapy

Both external radiotherapy and radio-iodine are usually given with radical intent although palliative treatment is occasionally justified, particularly external therapy for anaplastic tumours.

### Thyroid replacement

Marginally supra-physiological replacement, sufficient to cause TSH suppression below the normal range, can help control some advanced differentiated cancers.

### Cytotoxic chemotherapy

This has little place in the treatment of thyroid cancer other than lymphomas.

## Follow-up

Prolonged follow-up is justified for most patients since even widespread differentiated carcinomas can be eradicated with radio-iodine and the chance of eradication is higher the smaller the tumour burden. Recurrences of some indolent carcinomas can occur more than two decades after original treatment. As well as careful clinical examination of the neck, periodic whole body radio-iodine scans, chest X-rays and TSH estimations are justified for these patients. Serial estimations of serum thyroglobulin concentration can lead to the early detection of regrowth of some differentiated carcinomas following complete ablation of normal thyroid, since they release thyroglobulin into the circulation. Serial estimation of calcitonin is essential in the follow-up of patients treated for medullary carcinoma.

## Practice points

1 Indirect laryngoscopy must be performed prior to thyroid surgery to establish normal vocal cord movement.
2 Fine needle aspiration cannot reliably distinguish benign from malignant follicular neoplasms.
3 Patients with a familial history should have a serum calcitonin estimation pre-operatively.
4 All patients with known or suspected medullary carcinoma should have urinary catecholamine levels measured pre-operatively, since a phaeochromocytoma may co-exist (Multiple Endocrine Neoplasia Type II) and demand expert anaesthetic and peri-operative medical supervision.
5 Patients who have received ablative doses of radio-iodine must not be allowed home (or out of their hospital room) until their level of radioactivity has declined to a permissible level, usually a couple of days after administration. They should also be advised against sharing a bed or going near children during the immediate week or so after they return home, and should avoid attending public places of entertainment, long journeys on public transport, close contact with pregnant women and immediate return to work. They should restart thyroid replacement on discharge.

# NOTES

# Useful Addresses for Patients

Breast Care and Mastectomy Association of Great Britain
26 Harrison Street
King's Cross
London WC1H 8JG
Tel: 01-837 0908

British Association of Cancer United Patients (BACUP)
121–123 Charterhouse Street
London EC1M 6AA
Tel: 01-608 1661 (Cancer Information Service – 6 lines)
01-608 1785/6 (Administration)

Cancer Aftercare and Rehabilitation Society (CARE)
21 Zetland Road
Redland
Bristol BS6 7AH
Tel: 0272 427419
An organisation of patients, relatives and friends who offer help and support. There are branches throughout the country.

Cancer Link
46a Pentonville Road
London N1 9HF
Tel: 01-833 2451
Provides training and advice for people setting up support groups and a telephone information service.

Cancer Relief Macmillan Fund
15–19 Britten Street
London SW3 3TY
Tel: 01-351 7811
Provides home care nurses and financial grants.

Colostomy Welfare Group
38–39 Eccleston Square
London SW1V 1PB
Tel: 01-828 5175
Provides support and encouragement, free literature and information.

CRUSE
Cruse House
126 Sheen Road
Richmond
Surrey TW9 1UR
Tel: 01-940 4818
A national organisation for the widowed and their children. Offers a counselling service. Branches throughout the country.

Hodgkin's Disease Association
PO Box 275
Haddenham
Aylesbury
Bucks HP17 8JJ
Tel: 0844 291500
Publishes information and answers written and telephone enquiries. Puts people in touch with others who have had the disease.

Hysterectomy Support Groups
11 Henryson Road
Brockley
London SE1 1WL
Tel: 01-690 5987
Provides information about hysterectomy, and local hysterectomy support groups.

Incontinence Advisory Service
380–384 Harrow Road
London W9 2HU
Tel: 01-289 6111
Provides information and advice.


Marie Curie Memorial Foundation
28 Belgrave Square
London SW1X 8QG
Tel: 01-235 3325
Provides nursing homes and a community nursing service.


National Association of Laryngectomy Clubs
39 Eccleston Square
London SW1V 1PB
Tel: 01-834 2857
Provides patients with the opportunity to meet.


National Society for Cancer Relief
Michael Sobell House
30 Dorset Square
London NW1 6QL
Tel: 01-402 8125
Provides financial support to needy patients and their families.


Patients Association
18 Charing Cross Road
London WC2H 0HR
Tel: 01-240 0671


Stoma Advisory Service
Abbott Laboratories Ltd
Queenborough
Kent ME11 5EL
Tel: 0795 663371
Provides advice and publishes booklets.

Tak Tent
132 Hill Street
Glasgow
Tel: 041-332 3639
Provides training courses for people setting up support groups
and written information.

Tenovus Cancer Information Centre
11 Whitchurch Road
Cardiff CF4 3JN
Tel: 0222 619846
Provides counselling and information over the telephone.

Ulster Cancer Foundation
40–42 Eglantine Avenue
Belfast BT9 6DX
Tel: 0232 663281
Provides information over the telephone.

Urostomy Association
Buckland
Beaumont Park
Danbury
Essex CM3 4OE
Tel: 024541 4294

# Useful Publications for Patients

All are either free or of low or moderate price.

## Publications by BACUP (address above)

Cancer of the Bladder

Cancer of the Breast

Cancer of the Cervix

Cancer of the Colon and Rectum

Cancer of the Kidney

Cancer of the Lung

Cancer of the Oesophagus

Cancer of the Ovary

Cancer of the Pancreas

Cancer of the Prostate

Cancer of the Skin

Cancer of the Stomach

Cancer of the Testes

Cancer of the Thyroid

Cancer of the Uterus

Cervical Smears

Chemotherapy

Diet and the Cancer Patient

Hair Care

Hodgkin's Disease

Malignant Melanoma

Non-Hodgkin's Lymphoma

Radiotherapy

# Booklets in the Patient Information Series from the Patient Education Group, Royal Marsden Hospital

These can be ordered from:
Haigh and Hochland Ltd
International University Booksellers
The Precinct Centre
Oxford Road
Manchester M13 9QA
Tel: 061-273 4156

Breast Self-Examination

Cancer of the Bladder – Your Questions Answered

Cancer of the Breast – Your Questions Answered

Cancer of the Cervix – Your Questions Answered

Cancer of the Ovary – Your Questions Answered

Care of a Skin Tunnelled Catheter

Chemotherapy – Your Questions Answered

Clinical Trials

Coping with Cancer

Hysterectomy – Your Questions Answered

Laryngectomy – Your Questions Answered

Leukaemia – Your Questions Answered

Lung Cancer – Your Questions Answered

Lymphomas – Your Questions Answered

Overcoming Eating Difficulties – A Guide for Cancer Patients

Radiotherapy – Your Questions Answered

Testicular Self-Examination

# Other Useful Publications

A Patient's Guide to Chemotherapy
Pauline Hammond.
Available free of charge from Lederle Laboratories, A Division of Cyanamid of Great Britain Ltd, Fareham Road, Gosport, Hants PO13 0AS

All About Cancer – A Practical Guide to Cancer Care
Chris Williams.
Wiley, Chichester, 1983.

Breast Cancer – The Facts
Prof. M. Baum.
Oxford University Press, 1988.

Cancer: A Guide for Patients and their Families
Chris and Sue Williams.
Wiley, Chichester, 1986.

Cancer Self Help Groups Directory
Available from Cancer Link (address on page 341).

Cancer: What it is and How it is Treated
H. Smedley, K. Sikora and R. Stepney.
Basil Blackwell, Oxford, 1986.

Caring for the Very Sick Person at Home
Available from Cancer Link (address on page 341).

Cervical Cancer and Radiotherapy – Putting You in the Picture
A. K. Carr and Pauline Cornish.
Available free of charge from Lederle Laboratories, A Division of Cyanamid of Great Britain Ltd, Fareham Road, Gosport, Hants PO13 0AS

Chemotherapy: A Guide for Patients
Prof. J. M. A. Whitehouse.
Available free of charge from Farmitalia Carlo Erba Ltd., Italia House, 23 Grosvenor Road, St Albans, Herts AL1 3AW

Coping with Breast Cancer
Available from the Breast Care and Mastectomy Association of Great Britain (address on page 341).

Coping with Cancer: Making Sense of it All
Rachael Clyne.
Thorsons Publishing Group, Wellingborough, 1986.

General Information Pack for Mastectomy Patients
Produced by the Breast Care and Mastectomy Association (address on page 341).

Giving Up Smoking with the Help of Nicorette
A free booklet to accompany this proprietary brand of nicotine chewing gum.
Available from Lundbeck Ltd, Lundbeck House, Hastings Street, Luton, Bedfordshire LU1 5BE

Life with Cancer
Available free of charge to people with cancer and their families from the cancer support group Cancer Link (address on page 341).

Living with a Colostomy
M. Schindler.
Turnstone Press, Wellingborough, 1986.

Living with Cancer
Jenny Bryan & Joanna Lyall.
Penguin Books, 1987.

Living with Cancer
A leaflet published by the Wessex Cancer Trust.
Available free of charge from The Information Officer, Wessex Regional Cancer Organisation, Royal South Hants Hospital, Graham Road, Southampton SO9 4PE

Oral Morphine
Information for patients, families and friends.
Beaconsfield Publishers, 20 Chiltern Hills Road, Beaconsfield HP9 1PL

Understanding Cancer
Published by the Which? organisation. Consumers' Association, PO Box 44, Hertford SG14 1SH

Several publications on alternative medicine for cancer patients are listed in *What Your Patients May be Reading*, Robert Gann, British Medical Journal, **295**, 1273–1274, 1987.

# Index